ADHD PARENTING STRATEGIES

Everything You Need to Know to Stop Your Kids Anxiety, Improve Their Organization and Get Them Focused and Motivated

By Laurel Nash

© **Copyright 202x - All rights reserved.**

The content contained within this book may not be reproduced, duplicated or transmitted without direct written permission from the author or the publisher.

Under no circumstances will any blame or legal responsibility be held against the publisher, or author, for any damages, reparation, or monetary loss due to the information contained within this book, either directly or indirectly.

Legal Notice:

This book is copyright protected. It is only for personal use. You cannot amend, distribute, sell, use, quote or paraphrase any part, or the content within this book, without the consent of the author or publisher.

Disclaimer Notice:

Please note the information contained within this document is for educational and entertainment purposes only. All effort has been executed to present accurate, up to date, reliable, complete information. No warranties of any kind are declared or implied. Readers acknowledge that the author is not engaged in the rendering of legal, financial, medical or professional advice. The content within this book has been derived from various sources. Please consult a licensed professional before attempting any techniques outlined in this book.

By reading this document, the reader agrees that under no circumstances is the author responsible for any losses, direct or indirect, that are incurred as a result of the use of the information contained within this document, including, but not limited to, errors, omissions, or inaccuracies.

Remeber!

Listening is a primary skill to manage if you want to be a better parent.

Develope it by listening to the Free Audiobook version of this script!

Scan the QR code:

Summary

ADHD PARENTING STRATEGIES 1
INTRODUCTION 5
CHAPTER 1 9
   Basics of Adhd 9
CHAPTER 2 26
   Common myths about Adhd 26
CHAPTER 3 35
   The challenges of growing up with Adhd 35
CHAPTER 4 59
   Practical and loving parenting 59
CHAPTER 5 93
   Teaching your child self-care 93
CONCLUSION 121

INTRODUCTION

WHAT IS ADHD?

One of the most prevalent mental disorders affecting children is Attention-Deficit Hyperactivity Disorder (ADHD). Many adults are still affected by ADHD. Inattentiveness (the inability to stay focused), hyperactivity (being unusually or abnormally active), and impulsivity are all symptoms of ADHD (rash acts that occur in the minute without thought).

ADHD affects about 8.4% of children and 2.5 percent of adults. When ADHD causes disturbance in the classroom or difficulties with schoolwork, it is commonly diagnosed in school-aged children. Adults may be affected as well. It is more prevalent in boys than in girls.

What Does It Mean to Have ADHD?

Have you ever been asked if you have ADHD? Perhaps you've had similar thoughts. The best way to know for sure is to see a physician. This is because the disease may have a wide range of manifestations and can be easily associated with those of other disorders such as clinical depression or stress and anxiety.

Not sure whether a doctor should examine you? If you have

any of these symptoms, you should see a doctor.

1. People say you are absent-minded.

From time to time, everybody drops their car keys or jackets. When you have ADHD, something happens. Every day, you may be shopping for glasses, wallets, tablets, and a variety of other things. You may even refuse to answer phone calls, pay bills early, or cancel medical appointments.

2. People complain that you do not pay attention to.

Most of us lose focus on a conversation from time to time, particularly if there is a television nearby or something else vying for our attention. And when there are no distractions available, it happens frequently and more frequently in people with ADHD. Even now, ADHD is more than that.

3. You're typically behind schedule.

When you have ADHD, time management is a constant struggle. Unless you take steps to avoid it, it normally results in missing deadlines or appointments.

4. You have difficulty concentrating.

Interest issues, mostly concentrating on long stretches of time without paying attention to data, are only a few of the problem's characteristics. Depression, anxiety, and alcohol issues will also affect the ability to concentrate, and many people with ADHD suffer from one or more of these issues. Your doctor will help you figure out what's causing your concentration problems by asking you questions.

5. You leave things undone.

It can be difficult to start or finish projects if you have problems with interest or memory. Specifically, ones that you know would need a lot of focus to complete. This condition may also signify depression.

6. You had behavior concerns as a child.

And if those early symptoms didn't present an official diagnosis, you would have had concentration and concentrating problems as a child to be diagnosed with ADHD as an adult. People may have accused you of being lazy when you were younger. They may have assumed you had a secondary concern, such as depression or stress and anxiety. You could still have the disease if you were diagnosed as an infant. When you get older, the symptoms shift, and not everybody outgrows it.

7. You lack impulse control.

It's more than about throwing a candy bar into the shopping cart at the checkout counter. It's when you do something despite knowing it might have serious consequences, such as breaking a red light when you think you'll get away with it or otherwise being able to keep the peace because you have something to say, while knowing you should.

8. You cannot get organized.

You might learn more about this at work. Setting goals, keeping up on projects, and reaching project deadlines can be challenging for you.

9. You're nervous.

Adults with ADHD are more likely to be fidgety or troubled than children with ADHD. You may even speak too loudly or annoy someone.

10. You can't control your emotions.

You can be irritable or irritable, often show anger, feel indifferent, or be prone to violent outbursts. When you have ADHD, it can be difficult to cope with uncomfortable emotions or maintain good behavior when you are disturbed.

CHAPTER 1
Basics of Adhd

ADHD and Its Causes

Before we get through the different forms of ADHD symptoms, it's important to first understand what causes the disorder. There are a variety of factors that contribute to this problem. The majority of experts, however, believe that this neurodevelopmental disease is mostly a genetic disorder. We also have a part of our brain that is responsible for 'executive functioning.' When an infant suffers from ADHD, the area of the brain is affected. That is the primary explanation that all adolescents with this condition have difficulty expressing appropriate thoughts, planning their future, evaluating all of their actions, controlling hyperactive impulses, or solving problems. Because of the different forms of complications that can arise in any kind of family because of ADHD-related issues, it's easy to lose sight of the truth. If the issue worsens, it can have a negative impact on the child's school actions as well as their personal relationships.

Any parents claim that the issues arose because of a flaw in their parenting style. There are also those who believe that this neuro-developmental condition is the product of a traumatic incident that occurred in their child's life during their early years, or any painful or traumatic event that they were a part of. Teachers who are unaware of the problem or who fail to recognize the severity of the issue can mark the student as lazy or disobedient. However, if you really wish to assist someone who is suffering from this crisis, whether an adult or a child, you must first learn about the disorder's origins. It is true that a genetic factor plays a role in the development of ADHD. However, you must keep in mind that the blame should not have to be placed solely on the parents of a child with ADHD, since they are unable to change the situation.

- ADHD and Heredity

There is a group of parents who are all wondering the same thing: "Is ADHD genetic or not?" The response to this question is, of course, yes. ADHD is a genetic disorder. It may be classified as a common illness or condition that runs in families. A vast amount of research has been done over the past thirty years to learn more about ADHD. If you want to keep track, there have been over two thousand experiments completed to date. Researchers are doing their research to learn more about the true nature of ADHD. Psychiatrists, psychiatrists, and geneticists have also collaborated to learn more about this condition. Most of the time, a child with ADHD would have had someone in his or her family, whether it was their own parents or another blood relative, who already had ADHD.

Until now, various forms of genes have been discovered. All of them are most definitely linked to the illness. However, further research is also being done on this subject in order to better specify the precise genetic markers. If you know what has been discovered so far, it has been discovered that there isn't just one gene that is exclusively responsible for this. However, you should be aware that no genetic tests for ADHD have been performed to date. Often, there are several misconceptions because just because a person is genetically predisposed to having ADHD symptoms does not mean that he or she would. There have been many instances where children did not experience ADHD despite the presence of the condition in their families. There have also been occasions where children experience ADHD even though no one in their family has the condition. Since there is a genetic connection to ADHD, certain parents felt responsible for their child's condition because they think it was their fault.

It's also been discovered that when a family has a child with ADHD, approximately 25% of the family members exhibit the disorder's symptoms. In contrast to a family without someone suffering from ADHD, the prevalence is even higher. Furthermore, if a parent has identical twins and one of them has already developed ADHD signs, the odds of the other sibling having the condition are around 83 percent. If the twins are fraternal, the average ratio drops to 39 percent. All these figures clearly demonstrate the strong connection between ADHD and genetics.

• Anatomy of The Brain

More research is being conducted to determine the relationship between brain structure and ADHD. It has also been discovered that certain areas of the brain of children do not develop as well as others. Having said that, this should not imply that children with ADHD symptoms are not gifted or intelligent. To put it another way, certain areas of the brain take longer to completely mature. In terms of cognitive regulation and working memory, some of these mechanisms are critical. That is the predominant explanation why the self-management brain system suffers. However, by the time the afflicted infant enters maturity, all these vital structures have changed and are on their way to being fully developed.

You must comprehend that the way the brain works is comparable to turning gears. To write or read, all the related parts must work together. The neurons are the connections that serve to bind the different brain cells. Many of these neural networks take longer to mature while a child suffers from ADHD symptoms. One of these neural networks is designed to induce a resting period in the child. It's also known as the "default mode network." When a child with this condition, they are unable to focus well because the default mode network takes longer to place other aspects on hold or rest. The fronto-parietal network is another important pathway that is impacted. It is the network that facilitates a child's ability to discover and learn new things as well as take effective decisions.

- Other Related Factors

Children can develop ADHD in some cases if they sustain a head injury during their childhood. Some forms of parental exposure can be very dangerous to infants and can also lead to ADHD. Alcohol and nicotine are two examples of such exposures. There are a few instances where the troubling effects of ADHD are caused by environmental factors. When an infant is exposed to lead, for example, it often results in abnormal behavior and stunted development.

- Other Causes of ADHD

The reason your child has ADHD can be traced back to family members. The disorder is genetically dependent, which means your child could have been predisposed because of your genetics. And if conditions at home or at school worsen, they are not considered causes of ADHD.

Many scientific studies have linked physical features to the cause of ADHD. These factors include genetics, absorbing toxic active substances, brain trauma, and reactions to artificial additives.

- The Make-Up of Your Genetics:

Examine the other members of the family. Did you know that while only three to five percent of children are diagnosed with ADHD, 25 percent of an ADHD child's family are still diagnosed with the disorder? Specific genes have also been traced to the root cause of ADHD, according to scientific studies!

- Toxic Components:

Researchers also discovered a potential correlation between drinking alcohol or using tobacco products while pregnant and having an ADHD foetus. These toxic compounds would almost inevitably be absorbed by an embryo, which cannot be well. If your kid has been exposed to old homes, he may be suffering from lead poisoning. Several of these toxic additives have been linked to the development of ADHD. My father exposed me to DDT, which is now banned in the United States, while I was growing up on a farm. That may have contributed to my ADHD, and then my son's.

Fortunately, most children do not fall into this category;

however, some types of emotional trauma may cause ADHD symptoms. When an ADHD child and a non-ADHD child have brain scans or an MRI, there were certain differences in certain areas of the mind, according to scientific research. This may seem to indicate that the brain is involved in the cause of ADHD.

Food Additives: As sugar and additive consumption is decreased, about 10% of ADHD children show reduced symptoms. Right now, there's something unexpected. While all of us, including me, equate candy with attention deficit disorder, when children were given either sugar or a sugar substitute, there was no distinction. This means that sugar does not play a role in the symptoms of ADHD.

Given that many people believe that sugar causes ADHD symptoms, they can see more symptoms when a child consumes sugar. According to studies, parents who think their children have been given sugar (when they have been given a substitute) are about as likely to report that ADHD symptoms have increased as parents whose children have been given real sugar.

A decrease in sugar intake (or high fructose) may be helpful even though it is only considered.

Preservatives and food coloring, which can be used in soft drinks and fast food, have been found to greatly increase hyperactivity in children, according to a new report. As a result, make sure you're aware of what they're putting into their bodies.

Remember the ADHD causes children to behave in inappropriate ways. This isn't the only way to go about it. It is a very treatable condition. Prescription medications to target the symptoms, herbal therapies to target the cause of the problem, diet management, and behavioral treatment are all options. Do your research first, and then do what is best for your child.

• **Symptoms of ADHD**

As previously stated, the main signs of ADHD in children include impulsive and hyperactive behavior patterns. They're all primarily inattentive. The signs and symptoms of ADHD can be seen as early as childhood. Furthermore, the signs can be seen as early as three years of age. However, signs of the condition can appear at any time before the diagnosed child reaches the age of twelve. Let's take a look at some of the more common ADHD signs.

- Hyperactivity and Impulsivity

Do you have a kid that likes to be on the move all of the time? Is he/she always talking even when it isn't necessary? These are, after all, the most prominent signs of hyperactivity. When you see your kid repeatedly interrupting the worried questioner and answering any question when they are not meant to, you know they are impulsive. That can even happen when your child is impatient to get or do something. All children with ADHD have an unavoidable need to interrupt others' discussions, activities, and games. When they are asked to complete something quietly, they begin to exhibit signs of difficulty.

Children with ADHD are constantly fidgeting with their hands or feet. They squirm in their seats if they are asked to sit silently for a period of time. When you ask them to sit calmly in one position, they can start running or climbing around. It's possible that it's one of the main reasons that children with ADHD had so many difficulties in education. Another typical symptom is your child's intense focus on his or her own requirements or desires, to the point that they neglect or pay little heed to the needs of others. They may be in a constant state of upheaval. In addition, your child will find it difficult to place a buffer between his or her emotions. Yes, they can display a great deal of interest in a variety of topics. However, when it comes to completing them before moving on to the next, they simply try to miss the section and leave the job unfinished.

- Inattention

If you find that your kid is always making stupid mistakes in school or that he or she is not working hard enough to pay attention to even the smallest details, the odds are that he or she is inattentive. Another indication of being inattentive is when your child does not react appropriately when you are conversing with them directly. Additionally, the child can display signs that they are not entirely concentrated on the most basic activities during the day. Inattention can manifest itself in a variety of ways, including the child being readily diverted from the task at hand. They might also have a lot of trouble with organization. When your child tries to pull away their eyes from tasks that need them to remain focused, such as school homework, you can quickly determine that they are suffering from inattention. You can see the same thing in different circumstances where your child has a habit of losing valuable items that are needed for completing tasks or other important matters.

- The Various Types of ADHD

- Comprehending ADHD

Attention deficiency hyperactivity disorder (ADHD) is a long-term disease. It mainly affects infants, but it may also affect adults. It has an effect on feelings, attitudes, and learning abilities. There are three distinct forms of ADHD:

- Inattentive type

- Hyperactive-impulsive type

- Combination of both types

The type of ADHD you have can be determined by your signs and symptoms. Signs and symptoms of ADHD must have an effect on the everyday life in order to be diagnosed.

Because the signs and symptoms of ADHD may vary over time, the form of ADHD you have will also change. ADHD can be a long-term challenge. Medicine and a variety of other treatments will help you live a better life.

• Three Types of Symptoms

Several characteristics are associated with each form of ADHD. Inattentiveness and hyperactive-impulsive behavior are symptoms of ADHD.

These traits can be seen in all groups of people: Sidetrackedness, lack of focus, and management skills are also examples of inattentiveness.

Impulsivity: disturbing, risk-taking

Hyperactivity: never seems to slow down, talks while fidgeting, and has difficulty staying on track.

Since everybody is different, it's common for two people to

have different reactions to the same signals. These habits, for example, are common in both young boys and girls. Children may appear to be more hyperactive, and girls may appear to be silently unobservant.

• Inattentive ADHD

If you have this form of ADHD, you may see that you have a lot more signs and symptoms of inattention than impulsivity or hyperactivity. At times, you can struggle with impulse control or hyperactivity. This aren't the only prominent characteristics of inattentive ADHD.

People who experience inattentiveness commonly:

- Miss details and also are sidetracked quickly
- Get tired rapidly
- Have difficulty concentrating on a solitary task
- Have trouble organizing thoughts and also learning brand-new info
- Lose pencils, papers, or various other things needed to finish a task
- Don't appear to pay attention
- Move slowly and also look as if they're daydreaming

- Refine details much more slowly as well as much less appropriate than others

- Have a problem following directions

Women are diagnosed with inattentive form ADHD at a higher rate than men.

• Hyperactive-Impulsive ADHD

Signs of impulsivity and attention deficit disorder characterize this form of ADHD. This personality style may show signs of inattentiveness. It is, however, not as important as the other symptoms.

People that are impulsive or hyperactive frequently:

- Squirm, fidget, or feel restless

- Have difficulty sitting still

- Talk continuously

- Touch as well as play with objects, even when inappropriate to the task at hand

- Have trouble engaging in quiet tasks

- Are regularly "on the move"

- Are impatient

- Act out of turn and also don't think of repercussions of actions

- Spout out answers and also inappropriate remarks

Children with hyperactive-impulsive ADHD can cause disruption in the class. They are capable of doing more discovery tasks on their own than most students.

• Combination ADHD

If you have the mix kind, that means the signs and symptoms aren't all related to inattentive or hyperactive-impulsive actions. Instead, a combination of signs and effects from both groups is displayed.

Many people, whether they have ADHD or not, have uncontrollable or spontaneous behavior. Individuals with ADHD, on the other hand, are at a higher risk. The habits appear constantly and obstruct your ability to act at home, school, work, and in social interactions.

Most children have hybrid type ADHD, according to the Central Institute of Mental Health. Hyperactivity is the most frequent symptom in preschool children.

- **Diagnosis of ADHD**

Now that you are well aware of the symptoms, if you believe your child is exhibiting any of them, the time has come to meet with a general practitioner. If you're not sure if you're taking the right moves, consult your child's teachers. Try to find out whether they talk about the same symptoms that your child has at kindergarten. Your general practitioner may not be able to diagnose ADHD. However, choosing a general practitioner first is important. On your first appointment, your primary care physician might ask you some standard questions.

- What are the symptoms you've seen in your child recently? When did you first notice all of this?

- When do you think the signs are more likely to appear? Is it happening at home or at school?

- Is it difficult for him/her to socialize with others because of the symptoms? Is there anybody else in your family with ADHD?

- Have you found any other signs that you think are worth noting that aren't linked to ADHD?

Following your consultation with your general physician, he or she will encourage you to have your child under close supervision for a period of time. The time is typically between ten and eleven weeks. During this time, you will be able to determine whether or not your child has improved in some way. You'll also learn why the pre-existing conditions have been the same or have become worse. In certain cases, the general practitioner can also recommend parent preparation or a special education curriculum for children with ADHD. However, there is something that you must comprehend at this stage. When you're told you should get parent training, that doesn't mean it's just because of you or that you're a bad parent.

Its aim is to show you all of the techniques for dealing with your kid in a more effective manner and to help them change their current situation. If your symptoms haven't changed since this period, you'll need to get professional support with a standardized evaluation. If you consider what kind of expert you will be referred to, you will find that there are many who will assist you with your problem. It's possible that you'll be called to meet with all of them.

You might be asked to consult any of them-

- When it is about child health, you might be recommended to visit a pediatrician

- A child psychiatrist relying on the patient's age

- A social worker, occupational therapist, or a specialist in learning disability

The person to whom you are referring will differ based on your location and the patient's age. A single examination would never be enough to determine whether or not your child is suffering from ADHD issues. However, a thorough examination by a specialist in this field will certainly shed some light on the true situation. A variety of interviews with your child and you are some of the common facets of those assessments.

The results of a physical examination of the infected child will then be revealed.

Interviews with other people, such as family members, partners, and students, are also conducted.

However, there are certain defined requirements that must be met in order to correctly identify a teenager or infant with ADHD issues.

The signs began to appear just before the child turned 12 years old, and they have been constant for at least six months.

The symptoms make it very difficult for the infected child to lead a normal social and academic life.

The symptoms do not only appear in one area, but in two entirely different conditions. For example, at home and at school, so that the infected child's symptoms are not caused by the teacher's care or parental control.

CHAPTER 2

Common Myths About Adhd

In any aspect of life, there are misconceptions and myths, and ADHD is no exception. When myths and misconceptions become entrenched in society, however, the situation will quickly escalate into a big issue. People begin to believe them, and as a result, you will be unable to distinguish between true and false information. That is the primary explanation why disease-related misconceptions and myths will cause significant harm. As a result, it is important to dispel those misconceptions and examine the problem objectively. In addition, myths and misconceptions can make the recovery process tedious at times. In this part, we'll dispel some of the more common misconceptions about ADHD so you don't underestimate your child.

• ADHD Cannot Be Regarded as a Real Disorder

Most care practitioners, clinical and psychiatric specialists, and organizations and associations in the United States have long regarded ADHD as a severe condition. The American Psychiatric Association, the National Institute of Health, and the Centers for Disease Control and Prevention are only a few of the main associations. The lack of a proper evaluation that can truly diagnose ADHD is one of the key reasons that contributes to misconceptions or misunderstandings regarding the disorder's status. A medical expert or a doctor, much as for most severe medical problems, cannot simply validate the diagnosis of ADHD with imaging and laboratory tests.

While there is no standard examination for the diagnosis of ADHD, there are certain specific and consistent conditions that must be followed in order for the diagnosis to be made. These guidelines, along with a clear history and knowledge about the concerned person's habits, will be used by mental health professionals and doctors to make an accurate diagnosis.

Another significant aspect is that ADHD signs aren't necessarily well described. ADHD is based on a specific pattern of habits. For every point in our lives, we all have difficulty concentrating and paying attention. However, for those with ADHD, any of these conditions can be serious enough to interfere with everyday life. Symptoms of ADHD may also be mistaken for those of other illnesses. Before an ADHD diagnosis may be made, any undiagnosed or pre-existing medical issues must be recognized.

• ADHD Is Often Over-Diagnosed

The evidence is somewhat ambiguous in this regard. According to annual reports, the diagnosis of ADHD in children in the United States is on the rise. However, other severe disorders such as anxiety, depression, and autism are also on the rise, according to the study. In terms of ADHD in particular, some studies have shown that the disorder could be under-diagnosed in situations where the cumulative signs are less evident. Female children's ADHD can manifest in a different way, according to a popular example gathered from the data. Although female children with ADHD are less likely to exhibit hyperactive symptoms, they can also have considerable difficulty focusing and performing mental tasks. According to a number of studies, female children are less likely than male children to be diagnosed with ADHD and to undergo some type of therapy for it.

Other studies, however, indicate that ADHD is often over diagnosed, especially in boys. Male children's ADHD prevalence could be higher in part due to gender stereotypes; for example, boys are more likely to act out physically. Boys are often more likely to exhibit aggressive and ADHD symptoms, which increases the likelihood that their attitudes will be noticed by teachers, parents, and physicians. Cultural, social, and racial causes have been discovered to play a part in the disparities in ADHD care and diagnosis. According to a 2016 survey, white children were the most likely to be diagnosed with ADHD and undergo medication for the condition. While the results say over-diagnosis, the researchers suggest that under-treatment and under-diagnosis of Latino and African American children with ADHD could be a more accurate reading of the evidence.

Adult ADHD is also over-diagnosed, according to another study. Adults are often suggested to be afflicted with ADHD symptoms as a result of the medicalization of their normal personality traits and life experiences. Other forms of learning disorders or mental health problems are often misdiagnosed as ADHD signs in some circumstances. Overdiagnosis with ADHD carries the main risk of inappropriate therapy with stimulant drugs. While the associated medications may be an effective treatment for ADHD, they can be misused if given to someone who does not need them.

• ADHD Can Only Be Found in Children

To fully meet the diagnostic criteria, ADHD signs must be present before the age of seven years. However, some patients do not get a diagnosis until they are well into adulthood. It is not unusual for certain parents to be diagnosed with ADHD at the same time as their offspring. When an adult learns more about the disorder, they can begin to recognize the symptoms of ADHD, as well as the habits that go along with it, in themselves. When they reflect on their youth, they might remember that the difficulties they had in school were most likely the product of unresolved or overlooked concentration issues. A correct diagnosis at any time can sound like a relief to children and parents. It can be reassuring to be able to assign labels to symptoms while still recognizing that there are ways to effectively treat them.

Many children who are diagnosed with ADHD symptoms can continue to exhibit the symptoms as teens and adults. However, as the symptoms progress, the general meaning of the symptoms can alter. For example, the hyperactive aspect of typical children's habits seems to diminish with age. Distractibility, inattention, and restlessness, on the other hand, can continue into adulthood. Adult ADHD that is poorly treated will lead to long-term complications in relationships and at work. ADHD that goes untreated and undiagnosed has been attributed to drug abuse, depression, and anxiety.

• ADHD Is the Result of Bad Parenting

Parents of ADHD children should be concerned that they are to blame for their children's misbehavior. However, the overall situation is not solely due to poor upbringing. Any kid, whether or not they have ADHD symptoms, may be negatively affected by critical and punitive parenting or a disorderly household. Both of these causes can make it more difficult for children to deal with the effects of ADHD, but they are not the primary cause of the disorder. As a result, parents may want to reconsider their parenting style in order to best serve their ADHD infant. Children with ADHD have been shown to benefit from stable and straightforward outcomes and goals, as well as a predictable schedule at home.

- One of the Surest Symptoms of ADHD Is Hyperactivity

The word "attention deficit" in the name has led to misunderstandings about the overall meaning of the disease, as well as the perpetuation of numerous misconceptions about the symptoms. In reality, as we mentioned in the previous chapter, there are many forms of ADHD. Only the primarily hyperactive-impulsive type exhibits hyperactive habits, while the predominantly inattentive type does not. To avoid any misunderstanding, ADHD that is mostly inattentive is often referred to as attention-deficit disorder or ADD. Anyone exhibiting inattentive symptoms can be quickly distracted and daydreamy. They can even be forgetful, disorganized, and careless. This form of ADHD is often ignored. That is mostly due to the fact that it is less destructive than the hyperactive one. However, the associated effects may be very distressing for the person who is witnessing them all.

Although a child with ADHD is unlikely to outgrow the condition, some people describe developing out of hyperactive habits they had as children. Hyperactivity can be replaced by apathy and restlessness in some situations.

• People Suffering from ADHD Cannot Focus at All

Given the condition's name, seeing someone with ADHD/ADD intently focused on some task can be perplexing to certain people. Instead of being able to pay much attention, the portion of 'attention deficit' should be defined as trouble controlling focus. While people with ADHD have trouble planning, finishing, and working on tasks, it is not unusual for them to become completely involved in whatever things they find interesting. In fact, hyper-focus at this stage over an extended period of time may be a sign of ADHD.

• Stimulants Might Result in Addiction and Drug Abuse

There is a significant risk that stimulant drugs used to treat ADHD symptoms will lead to drug abuse. However, studies have shown that if ADHD is not treated, it will increase a person's chance of developing a drug use disorder. Untreated ADHD can also lead to depression or anxiety. To medicate their symptoms of ADHD and any other secondary nature of the psychological condition, a person can abuse illicit and licit drugs. It has since been discovered that people who undergo adequate ADHD therapy have a reduced rate of drug abuse, including stimulant medication.

• Medication Can Completely Treat ADHD

ADHD symptoms are not curable by medication. When administered under the supervision of a mental health specialist, it can easily assist with the management of symptoms. ADHD is a debilitating illness that will last a lifetime. If anyone is given ADHD treatment as a child, they will be required to take it as an adult as well. People can continue to experience the same symptoms as children as adults. Over time, the symptoms can diminish or simply improve. Both of these variations can be explained in part by developmental changes in the brain. They might also be a representation of how someone has learned to cope in the past.

Individuals with ADHD can learn organizational skills and coping strategies to help them cope with their symptoms. They will simply extend and continue to develop more of these abilities throughout their lives. They can also want to do it in conjunction with medications.

- ADHD Develops When Children Are Lazy

ADHD is not caused by a lack of ambition or laziness, but it should be considered a proper means of demeaning the actual problem. It's a genuine medical issue that needs to be treated. When a child has ADHD signs, he or she is not unable to concentrate on something. In fact, they are making every effort to do so. They would not, though, be able to do that. If you're just yelling at your kid to focus harder or being mean or mad at them that they aren't trying, it's pointless. It's akin to being enraged at others when they can't see anything because they're truly blind. The main factor attempting to influence your child's attentive capacity is not his or her personality. It is just due to certain physical differences in their brain that they are unable to do or do anything in the same way as most children. It's foolish to expect them to perform or behave like the other children because they aren't really made that way.

In reality, there are certain situations where parents do not fully comprehend the idea of ADHD and fault their children for not being able to concentrate or behaving in a certain manner. All of which seems to exacerbate the child's problems while still making him or her feel bad. When your kid has ADHD, you may need to create a large amount of prompts to get them to complete a mission. That does not, however, imply that your child is a slacker. All it means is that they lack the mental capacity to devote too much time. Even a simple game of building blocks may be mentally exhausting for a child suffering from ADHD symptoms. So, if you can only avoid blaming or comparing them for falling behind other children, it would be easier for them.

CHAPTER 3

The Challenges of Growing Up with Adhd

Children with ADHD, like all children, can be charming, playful, and creative. Children with ADHD are often more inventive and high-spirited than their peers, as well as more dynamic and creative. As a result, they have a plethora of plans and ventures in the works, and if their parents and teachers recognize their abilities and creative spirits, they can be very entertaining and enjoyable to be around. You've already seen this side of your child's personality and can enjoy the moments when all seems to go smoothly.

Childhood, on the other hand, can be difficult for anybody at times, and it can be especially difficult for children with ADHD. This children may struggle to keep up with their peers or, on the other hand, may outperform them in certain ways while falling behind in others. Children with ADHD mature at a slower rate than their peers, according to scientific research, but this does not suggest they will never catch up. That also doesn't suggest they're unaware of the disparities that distinguish them from their classmates, who might be rewarded and applauded more often at home and at school for socially appropriate conduct.

Children with ADHD may seem "out of it" at times; although they may seem unconcerned about their performance or actions, they are also painfully aware of their perceived shortcomings and sincerely desire to improve. Despite this, they also face developmental challenges that make it impossible for them to improve their behavior at school and at home without interventions and strategies adapted to their unique mental processes. As a consequence, without the proper assistance, they could develop a lack of self-confidence and an excessively negative perspective.

Although and child's journey is unique, many children with ADHD do not receive recognition for their abilities in traditional schools or at home. They can find it difficult to keep track of their possessions, complete their homework, remain silent while others talk, be tactful, and stay on task while doing chores, as their parents, family, and teachers expect. Their rooms may be disorganized, and their backpacks may resemble the effects of a blast. They can seem disobedient on purpose, but many of them crave adult approval.

Many children with ADHD have the feeling that if their parents and teachers took the time to notice their creative conversation, poetry, or skyscraper design, they would be considered talented. So, while your child's room may seem to be a disaster zone, underneath the chaos may be a very creative model plane, a stack of drawings, or a guitar and a stack of song lyrics they wrote themselves. Of course, these are all examples, so remember the likelihood that there are unexpected discoveries to be made about your boy. While it's true that children with ADHD have real talents waiting to be discovered, they often face common difficulties that aren't necessarily overlooked, such as the following:

ADHD Children's Common Challenges

- Problems following directions:

Children with ADHD also fail to obey instructions. They have trouble following oral instructions due to impulsivity or inattention, and they hardly read written directions carefully. They may seem to be daydreaming instead of listening and stubborn, despite the fact that they may truly wish to comply.

- Problems keeping track of belongings:

Children with ADHD have trouble keeping hold of their belongings at a much younger age than their peers. These children's parents may grow tired of buying them new mittens, backpacks, notebooks, and phones.

- Problems keeping track of time:

Children with ADHD also have a bad sense of time. Children with ADHD may be inefficient and lack a rational understanding of time, while most children tend to instinctively internalize how long it would take them to complete a job and how to arrive on time. As a result, they may rush through tasks carelessly or devote far too much time to a task, resulting in inefficiency.

- Difficulty getting started on tasks:

Initiating activities is one of the most complicated and difficult challenges for many children with ADHD to tackle. They can procrastinate for so long that they either do not begin tasks at all or have to hurry through them. Perfectionism frequently goes hand and hand with a child's trouble with initiation; in other words, these kids don't start assignments or practice well enough ahead of time to get a decent score, but they often have an unrealistic and urgent desire to complete these tasks completely, maybe to silence their own internal critic and the critics they encounter.

- Difficulty completing tasks:

Children with ADHD are more likely to get lost while

completing multi-step tasks. Starting the task, remaining focused, performing each mini step involved in the task, finishing the task, and turning their attention to the next step will all be difficult for them.

- A need for stimulation and activity:

Although a love of activity can help children become explorers and athletes, it can also make them uneasy at school, in places of worship, or in other formal environments. Furthermore, their desire for continuous stimuli may cause them to act rashly or rudely on occasion.

- Frustration:

Children with ADHD may get depressed when they make mistakes and believe they are not working up to their full potential. It can be difficult for these children to process feelings of discontent as they still have trouble managing their moods and rage. They can lash out at others around them at times.

- Low self-confidence:

Although certain children with ADHD can seem to have an unrealistically high degree of self-confidence (because they don't always have a clear idea of what they can fairly accomplish), they may be experiencing feelings of inferiority and self-worth as a result of their inability to keep up with tasks that are simpler for their peers. And if their parents and teachers compliment them, they tend to intuitively recognize that they are different (even if they don't realize they have ADHD), and they sometimes feel like they don't measure up.

- Social problems:

Since their impulsivity can involve an inability to censor their language and consider their behavior, some children with ADHD fail to sustain socially acceptable conduct. As a consequence, they may find it difficult to fit in with their peers.

- Academic problems:

At school, inattention and hyperactivity can lead to behavioral and academic issues. These shortcomings can be more pronounced in a typical school environment that prioritizes sitting still and doing rote writing work over individual speech. In these situations, children with ADHD get bored and act out to ease their boredom.

- Problems with mood:

Separate coexisting mood conditions, such as anxiety, depression, and bipolar disorder, are common in children with ADHD.

- Trouble with sleep–wake cycle:

Children with ADHD can have trouble sleeping at night and remaining awake throughout the day, causing them to appear and feel tired at school.

The Five Reinforcements for ADHD Behavior

Young children are obviously self-centered. They are vulnerable, and they depend on others for protection and assistance. The ability to command the attention of their caregivers is critical to their survival. Many hyperactive or impulsive patterns need motivation as well: these actions seem to attract others and cause situations to happen quickly.

As children get older, it is expected that they can gain more self-control and adhere to a greater number of laws. They continue to resent the limitations on their behavior. As a means of escaping responsibility for "big kid," inattention can be exacerbated at this time. In other words, behavior associated with ADHD (hyperactivity, impulsivity, and inattentiveness) will result in consequences that relieve the infant's distress. They will even persuade you and others to give your child more care and support. You should change the consequences of ADHD behavior and lessen the occurrence until you understand what strengthens the behavior. You will assist your child in developing new behaviors that have less harmful side effects and yield positive results.

- **The "Five A's"**

Your child's ADHD behavior may have one or more of the following positive outcomes: it may draw attention to her, it may persuade others to accommodate her, it may help her escape such circumstances, it may assist her in obtaining anything she desires, and it may persuade others to do something she dislikes. Any of the five "A"s will increase the incidence of ADHD behavior. These reinforcements may also be used in tandem to drive particular patterns and strengthen them even more.

- **Attention**

Your child can become rambunctious as soon as you start talking to a friend. This could be when your child is insecure because of your friendship with someone else. As soon as the focus is diverted away from her, they will try to attack off-limits items or make a noise. Such habits have the significant effect of causing you to be aware of what they are doing. Often what it takes is a familiar gesture or facial reaction for her to try to imitate this type of ADHD behavior.

ADHD behaviors can be an important way to keep a child focused. It's difficult to distance yourself from your daughter when she's distracted, hyperactive, insane, annoying, or distracting. Putting things close to your head or flopping around on your lap while talking to someone can be an efficient way to keep your mind going.

At school or at home, off-task tasks will draw a lot of scrutiny. Others may feel obligated to call your daughter and stay with her until she complies if she is floundering, fiddling, or not following orders. This will show her that other people care for her and are worried for her well-being. Her neglect can contribute to opportunities for support and motivation, and she may like it when someone calls her by her name or begs for a response. Her antics might also get her a seat next to you or her instructor.

Since the child has a target audience, waiting rooms and other public spaces are fertile ground for activity that draws attention. If you pass the time by reading a magazine, this ADHD behavior will emerge easily. Your daughter isn't malicious; she just wants to keep you engaged. Being loud and wild has a lot of disadvantages. The loudest and strangest person in the audience is usually the one who gets the most attention. Shouting can increase the likelihood of a response; clowning can be entertaining, and as people listen, parents find it more difficult to enforce limits.

People might argue that your child lacks the ability to "hold back" as much as others, but we can't forget the consequences of extreme behavior. This is particularly noticeable when the infant is speaking and thinking aloud.

They don't feel alone because of the relentless conversation, and you already wonder what she's up to when you hear a running joke. You're both related thanks to her chat and noise source. She will veer off on tangents, but no one else is allowed to speak about her never-ending story.

The stress caused by publicity-generating activity leaves no space for others. This does not actually imply that your child is receiving insufficient care. This clearly means that care is critical, and some children need greater assistance than others. When the family gathers together later in the day, practical jokes and multiple transgressions at school will usually make your kid the hot subject. And going against your will ensure that she is at the top of your priority list.

- **Accommodation**

When loved ones hear a child whine or cause difficulties, they also provide consolation. This may occur when your child overreacts, expresses frustration, is self-critical, or engages in any number of behaviors that indicate distress. When an infant is diagnosed with ADHD and deemed disabled, the people in their life are most likely to lower their expectations and provide help.

Social housing is also a result of ADHD behavior. If your kid makes a mess when she needs you to go, for example, rushing along will unintentionally increase her impatience. If your kid makes you get something extra to quiet her down, she will get more as a result of her bad behavior. And if you threaten to discipline her, she will continue to learn not to cooperate until you invest more time and resources. ADHD will motivate you to give more, do more, and work better than ever.

When your child is inattentive and depends on you to tell her what's going on, this is an example of this dilemma. She never learns to look after herself. If she does this at school, she is unlikely to graduate. Her teachers won't be able to keep up with her all of the time.

Joy and rescue can be linked in your child's mind. When she finds herself in a tough or risky situation, your efforts to protect her will serve as a reminder to her that she is important to you. And this entails checking and educating her about her specific self-care requirements.

The accommodating child also inquiries about issues that she can quickly resolve on her own. She adores the fact that you abandon everything in order to solve her problems. If you have reservations about her results, it would be difficult to impose conditions, hold her honest, or inspire her to help if you play foolish or dumb. Her ineffectiveness will make you worried about her, and it is your responsibility to help her through her difficulties. When you didn't mess with her, she complains, "Why have you not told me?" When you and others "take up the slack," she becomes unqualified as a result.

Your daughter will learn to be self-gratifying if she is used to being the object of your needs and worries at the expense of others. If she is used to endless pampering, she would be unable to adapt to what others crave. Showering her with concessions during the day or rewarding her with minor successes (such as going to the bathroom) can make it difficult for her to cope in circumstances where accommodations are scarce.

All of this means that ADHD activity is unlikely to decrease as long as social housing is severe. A child with ADHD behavior, like Paul's, can take over a household.

- **Paul's Story**

Paul was reluctant to consider or recognize his family's efforts to appease him. They were desperate to be successful parents because they came from homes with a large number of children. They put in a lot of effort to impress their family, as well as Paul. Paul, on the other hand, was not going to tell them he was happy. He didn't want to be obligated to give them up, and his parents worked even harder while he scowled. Paul kept hold of his family by letting them sound like losers, and he wouldn't let them off the hook. When Paul was angry, he became irritable and violent towards his younger brother, so his parents went to great lengths to ensure he wasn't upset. On times, he would sabotage an operation that did not suit his standards, and his parents would scramble to make it right.

They were frequently thinking about him during the day. They even planned their life to avoid bothering him. Despite their best attempts, he started to whine until pout, and he discovered that if he didn't quit, his parents would cave. When his parents were at their wit's end and calling out to him, he acted like a victim, and his parents feel guilty at the end of the day for losing their composure.

Unfortunately, Paul was disappointed that other people did not treat him as well as his parents did, and this became a major issue when he entered school. People didn't bend over backwards to appease him because of his hot temper and failure to change in that environment; instead, his habits caused him constant trouble. Since he was used to substantial accommodations at home, he was not sufficiently equipped to act in a classroom setting. He hadn't yet mastered the art of perseverance, avoided deception, or made an attempt to keep people happy.

Paul, predictably, chose not to complete his tasks. He would always leave incomplete tasks and projects and completing a small school job would take him hours. To save him from struggling and to calm the drama, his parents stayed with him and did all of the work for him.

Although Paul appreciated the fact that he was able to get his parents to help him with much of his homework, the disadvantage of this arrangement is clear: he did not meet his own standards. He just got good grades because his parents worked too hard. His parents really tried to support him, but he still picked up on a number of habits that were suggestive of an ADHD disorder.

Why Parents Over Accommodate

Parents will sometimes make accommodations on behalf of their children for a variety of reasons. Parents may believe that not protecting their children is too dangerous. If parents are concerned about future threats, they are more likely to take precautions. If they are vulnerable to embarrassment, they are often more likely to compromise. Single parents, in particular, may over-accommodate out of shame after a divorce, whether they believe they have failed the child because they have worked so many hours, or because the child has suffered the abandonment of the other parent.

Any parents are willing to please their children because of their own childhood poverty. These parents do not want to go through what their child has been through. Some are well suited to relieving the suffering of a traumatized infant. They deliberately solve problems so that the child does not face needless obstacles or risks. Some parents may go beyond for their children because they are in a hurry and don't have time to let them learn from their own mistakes. Some people are worried that they aren't good enough, and they are overjoyed to be accepted. And others assume the majority of the family's responsibilities because they were forced to do so as children. Whatever the reason or justification, compromise can stifle a child's ability to control his or her emotions and reach others halfway.

We also want to make it better for our children, but they must also understand that fighting is an inevitable part of life. Of course, striking a balance between too much anticipation and too little settlement is challenging. Although doing something pleasing to your daughter may help you develop a bond with her, you may also be encouraging acts that prevent her from working without your approval. As parents, we want our children to feel attached to us, protected, and cared for, but we also want them to establish self-reliance so that they can take care of themselves while we are not there. You are being supportive when you ease a project or send clues to a solution before making a fair attempt, but she does not want to exert herself.

Without your prompting, she will not learn to remember her belongings when you ask her to remove them. And, though offering to assist her with her dress saves time and makes it easier, it also delays the moment when she needs to properly put on her hat. In reality, you would create a lot of stress for yourself and learn to despise this system in the future.

- **Avoidance**

Avoidance is a natural way for both children and adults to deal with hardship. Distractibility, loss of concentration, and inability to listen, both of which are hallmarks of ADHD, may be perpetuated by avoidance advantages. "Staying out is better than going out," as Mark Twain once said. We don't gain control, though, so we disregard it, and the issue remains unanswered. Finally, neither of us can safely hide our heads in the sand like an ostrich.

Many adults no longer want to interpret a child's behavior as an inability to cooperate, join, or respond after he or she has been diagnosed with ADHD. They come to the conclusion that her ADHD prevents her from paying attention as we speak to her. They believe she won't be able to remember to slow down and pay attention to what you're doing. They assume she is hyper-focused pathologically if she wants to play and does not respond to your demands. People will consider thinking she hates you and now blame her ADHD for her lack of courtesy and sensitivity.

All of these distracted reactions, however, have advantages. These will also keep your daughter safe while also encouraging her to continue with her quest. She may believe that people are not listening to her, so she avoids listening herself. When people are negative or demanding, which means zoning out or yawning at them. When they force her to talk those subjects, she changes the subject. It even entails daydreaming and failing to acknowledge people.

Instead of being unable, your child may have learned that if she doesn't respond, she is exempt from the condition you impose. She has more time to do what she wants when she is easily distracted. It enables her to be carried away by her imagination.

Distractibility protects an infant from all types of suffering. It frees her from the constraints of assessment, punishment, and restraint. Her engrossment in her own thoughts and acts keeps her from engaging in unpleasant behaviors, such as those that are too simple or repeated.

Your kid may become lethargic and a tired look may sweep over her eyes as soon as she senses you nagging or lecturing her. Many people understand how difficult it is to listen to long speeches without receiving input. Many people can become arousal if the speech continues long enough, and their brain biology may mirror how they react. In children with ADHD, these types of responses occur often and quickly.

Your child may seem incapable, distracted, and confused, yet she's still ignoring and running from what bothers her because she doesn't have to learn something derogatory about herself or likely be disappointed. She may be much less likely to immerse herself and continue on the job if she knows she must be perfect or thinks others will appreciate her efforts. In these circumstances, even the tiniest noise in the room will spark her attention, even though it might go unnoticed at other moments where she is focused on her task.

Perhaps your daughter has a habit of not comprehending what she has just heard. It's natural if she drifts away staring at the phrases if she doesn't like what she's listening (or if she's worried about something else). And maybe, when she admits she can't concentrate, you'll stop chastising her and pressuring her to accomplish this kind of tedious mission, and then your efforts will seem pointless.

Fidgeting of things and squirming may also be symptoms of stress and a need to get away. Such behaviors often indicate that a child is disturbed by the situation and wants to flee. She may insist on not being able to remain in her current place but sitting in the corner and sharpening her pencil for an eternity allows her to put off the job she doesn't want to do for a long time.

Your child's play time would be increased if they do not organize their tools and do not complete their activities. She no longer puts it off because of the extra work and avoids unwanted events. If you challenge her, she can actually master new evasion techniques. When you challenge her to listen, she can chat or move, and you can't get a word in edgewise.

It's possible that "impulsive" behaviors are linked to avoidance. When she is disturbed, she can, for example, create a ruckus by acting rashly. She not only gets to let off steam, but she also effectively distracts her attention away from what is bothering her.

When your kid wanders around, rambles, and entertains you, you get a similar benefit. While acts can cause us to become more alert, they can also distract us from what is going on. This will effectively reduce family feuds or awkward silences. Your child's actions will assist with reducing stress levels.

- **Acquisition**

Many of the behaviors associated with ADHD cause a child to complete tasks more quickly. The proverbs "Strike while the iron is high" and "Take it while you can" illustrate the benefits of taking action quickly. Since it's difficult for someone to obstruct rapid and ambitious goal-oriented acts, such as going on to get the largest slice of cake, the kid who behaves quickly sometimes doesn't lose out. Others would be discouraged from denying anything they intend to refuse the child because of any ADHD behaviors. Your daughter can quickly get what she desires if her actions are unexpected, and she will want to give her change to others.

We don't like it when children choose, harass inappropriately, behave rudely, act recklessly, or cause harm on others, but it's difficult to break these habits when they perform too well. Your child will ping-pong around the house looking for something to do, much as you do while channel surfing. In general, ADHD behavior will help your child achieve happiness faster by speeding up the process and breaking downside barriers. Others are unable to anticipate their actions as a result of impulsive behavior, preventing them from obtaining what they want.

By blurring out what others are ashamed to reveal, your child can develop a sense of prestige. It's not that she lacks a filter; it's just that her actions, whether you like them or not, amplify her effect. They attempt to foster respectful conduct, but a child loses out less often when she is impolite, because it's often easier to say "sorry" than to ask for permission. They may believe the child lacks the ability to delay gratification or to be concerned about it before acting out, but it's simply her ADHD behavior that is too effective.

Even if unpleasant effects will follow, your daughter can love the thrill of having what she wants. When people rescue or smooth it out when there are potential complications, the deeds become much more important. Before assuming that her rashness is a sign of illness, it's crucial to figure out how often people save her.

- **Antagonism**

When your child is angry or upset, she may try to retaliate. Although certain children assertively or deliberately defend themselves in the face of conflict, children with ADHD are typically more discreet. They could, for example, throw small items in your face or play carelessly with a household piece. We call these acts impulsive, but they have a reason. They irritate you to no end, which is great for the kids.

The bigger the reaction to behavior, the more exasperated and irritated you are, the more likely the conduct will be repeated. Your kid will master the art of "pushing the buttons." When your kid is angry that he has to wait for an appointment, for example, his humiliating behavior will endanger you. You may think she's blurring out because she can't contain her emotions, but this isn't the case. By dragging her along, you can be depressed in a strong way.

It's not as if she's had difficulty "putting on the breaks." She baits and disrupts you if she makes a scene. She will flail about and repeatedly touch what you have forbidden her to touch. Both of these actions can be annoying, and they can even be used as a form of retaliation. She realizes you're bothered about your misbehavior in front of people, but she reminds you to be careful when you don't want to be labelled a poor mom. What is the source of your child's enmity?

The replies I've already provided suggest that there are already unresolved partnership problems. If you want to be a good father, you must first recognize and address these issues. You want your child to be able to cope with failure and confrontation successfully. Antagonism only serves to prolong the conflict.

Your girl, on the other hand, might not always be aware of what is worrying her. She may be instigating and frustrating you by realizing what she's mad over, and you may not know it. She may not be upset at you all of the time. Since you're either "clean" or the first one available, she could vent her frustrations on you. She will become enraged with you if you don't pay attention to her or fail to comply with her requests.

It's not always possible to figure out why a child is hostile. Relationships can be difficult to untangle. There are certain situations that bring up reminders of past events and disrupt your child's present relationship.

When a child overreacts, it can indicate that the problem has occurred on several occasions. It's difficult for everyone to cope with problems that keep happening, and your child can overreact in these situations. For example, if you've had a long-running disagreement, she may become unbearable because she thinks you're implying she's untrustworthy.

When your child perceives that you are unable to involve her, she will become hostile to you. Her obnoxious behavior may be a strategy for achieving superiority and escaping the disappointment that comes with being sweet. If she feels unwelcomed, she will retaliate by being rude. This will put pressure on you to adapt, and you will struggle as a result. "Misery likes business," as we all remember. Rather than getting teased and vulnerable, your child should do the hurting. When you're bothered or disgusted, she controls the rejection.

Antagonizing her can make her feel less alone, and it can also test whether you care enough to help her conquer her sadness and calm down. Antagonizing can also be hidden and circumvented. Your child will inform you that she will finish an assignment, but she may not. She might do a bad job on the assignment, lose it, or fail to turn it in. Many children with ADHD battle silently by struggling to complete tasks that are vital to their parents, such as schoolwork and household chores. Their weapon is failing, and they will now carry out their parents' worst fears. The battle, on the other hand, almost never yields positive results. Your child is becoming increasingly vulnerable, whilst you are becoming increasingly distressed.

CHAPTER 4
Practical and Loving Parenting

Parenting an ADHD child necessitates flexibility, innovation, and patience, not just with your child but also with yourself. If you can use the solutions discussed in this book to support your child, it is important to remember that ADHD needs long-term management. Yes, the symptoms will change, but the condition will not disappear immediately. It may be a chronic disease in some circumstances. Consider becoming a parent of a child with ADHD as a thrilling experience filled with many challenges, opportunities, and pleasant surprises!

Take, for example, Mariah, a physician. Mariah found it difficult to grasp and empathies with her child, Jackson, who was diagnosed with ADHD. He was obviously brilliant, but he did not do the job that was demanded of him and struggled in middle school. He discovered the wonder of physics in high school and excelled in the subject because he knew it too well. About the fact that Mariah did not always share Jackson's interests, she recognized and understood that he would do things differently than she had.

Although Mariah went straight to medical school after graduation, Jackson chose to work as an organic farmer in rural Maine for many years. He took pre-med classes at the same time, and after graduating from college, he enrolled in a science research degree programme. Along the way, he met a diverse group of people, learned how to plant, and applied real-world experience to his science studies.

Many children with ADHD, including Jackson, make unexpected decisions. Parents who remain agile and open-minded, on the other hand, will encourage and direct their children while they seek new talents and interests.

- When Parents Also Have ADHD

If you have ADHD, it can be much more difficult to parent your child with ADHD, but your experiences may help you to be more sensitive and receptive to what your child is going through. The world of ADHD has evolved dramatically in recent years. There is a clearer explanation of the disorder, as well as strategies, drugs, and other therapies that assist children with ADHD in doing well at school and at home. And, since far more children are correctly identified today than in previous years, they will get the assistance they need.

Any people with ADHD were not diagnosed when they were younger, and they may have grown up not knowing ADHD or making others realize what they were going through. If you identify with this, keep in mind that your child's experiences would most certainly vary from yours; now, there is a better awareness and acceptance of ADHD. You don't have to be concerned that your child's perceptions would mirror yours. Self-reflection is beneficial, but you should stop transferring any negatives from your experience into your kids. While the situation is the same, each individual is unique.

If you have ADHD as a child, you are obviously more sensitive to your child's difficulties and experiences. You should already be conscious that possessing the disorder has advantages. In reality, you should test out and develop techniques to support your child using your own sense of creativity and versatility.

- **Parenting Principles**

There are a few principles to bear in mind when you work with your child to create techniques for dealing with ADHD. These guidelines will assist you in guiding your child in a practical and compassionate manner, while also acknowledging that there is no treatment for ADHD. Your advice will assist your child in functioning at their own pace toward learning and dealing with the disorder.

Practice tolerance: Both parents need patience, but parents with children with ADHD need it even more so. While it is understandable for parents to try to "solve" their children's problems and "cure" their ADHD, the truth is that most children need time to mature. Children with ADHD progress in comparable ways to their peers, according to studies done by the NIMH and others, with the exception of brain growth, where they fall behind by around three years. According to these findings, parents should be confident that their children can learn the requisite organizational, organizing, and decision skills that children without ADHD do. However, because of the slower rate of maturation, extra maturity, and a focus on long-term growth, rather than fast fixes, could be needed.

Keep an eye on the long term: This is similar to patience. Parents should be aware that, through their efforts to assist their kids, they will not see instant results. Change and maturation take time, and children mature at different rates in different environments. They will face challenges along the way, but these setbacks do not mean they will not ultimately have any of the resources they need to live a full and prosperous life.

Ask others for help: While it is common for parents to try to support their children on their own, raising all children, especially those with intellectual disabilities, really "takes a village." In other words, get guidance and help from a group of people who have children with ADHD, whether online or in your neighborhood. Enlisting the assistance of people your child communicates with, such as instructors, mentors, tutors, physicians, therapists, and faith figures, is a good indicator of your parenting style. Enlisting the assistance of others can be especially necessary when your child approaches puberty, a time where children are less sensitive to what their parents have to offer.

Externalize rewards: As ADHD specialist Russell Barkley, PhD, points out in his book Taking Charge of ADHD, children with ADHD may not be able to internalize motivation as much as other kids over time, and they may need external motivation and encouragement to improve their behavior. This should not imply that parents should bribe their children; rather, parents should understand what desires children with ADHD have, such as computer games or sports, and use these interests as incentives for their children's fulfilment of more boring tasks. Although many parents wish their children to complete activities simply because they are the best thing to do, children with ADHD will need additional motivation before they acquire a more inherent understanding of what they need to do over time.

External incentives are suggested in some techniques in this book to keep your child focused.

Recognize positive behaviors: Children with ADHD are often in need of continuous reinforcement. Recognize what your child does right, even though it's just a little part of a bigger undertaking or something insignificant. Although most school-aged children will dress themselves and eat breakfast on their own, certain children with ADHD need encouragement for any part of the process they perform individually, such as putting on their socks or fixing their shoes without assistance or staying at the table for ten minutes without fidgeting. Although certain parents believe that children should not be congratulated for activities that are required of them at a certain age, children with ADHD need praise to keep them motivated to complete certain tasks independently. It may seem odd to applaud children who are still learning skills that their peers have mastered or that parents believe are easy, but it is important to keep children with ADHD on the path to independence. Big changes will happen in surprising ways, and little changes happen all the time; be unconditionally proud of your child and note when they excel, no matter how insignificant the achievement can seem to you.

Break down longer tasks and instructions into smaller, more manageable chunks: Children with ADHD often need longer tasks and directions broken down into smaller, more manageable chunks. Parents, therapists, and other providers do not assume that a child with ADHD would be able to break down more difficult activities on their own. For example, your child will need a list of all the tasks they must do in the morning. As an example, consider the following:

(1.) Take your clothes out of your drawer.

(2.) Put on your clothes starting with your socks, etc.

Similarly, school assignments must be broken down. And, since many children with ADHD lack an innate understanding of how to schedule or accomplish projects within a given time period, specific completion dates must be assigned.

Communicate with teachers and other professionals: Tell your child's teachers and other adults who deal with him or her, such as camp counsellors, the reality. Children with ADHD have a fundamental entitlement to special school accommodations, such as an Individualized Education Program (IEP), to assist them in succeeding. Many parents, though, try to hide an ADHD diagnosis for fear of their child being stigmatized. Teachers and those in teaching and caregiving positions may believe a child is being willfully disrespectful or destructive if they are unaware of the diagnosis. This insight will help teachers work for your child if you talk frankly about what your child is going through. Parents do not request that their children be excused from duties. Instead, they can consult with teachers to figure out ways to help their child finish his or her schoolwork.

Avoid comparing children to others, including siblings: Comparing children with varying needs and developmental trajectories to siblings or peers can be daunting. Children with ADHD often have a strong feeling of not matching up, and certain kinds of similarities do not help to inspire them when expressed with them. Using comparisons to teach a child with ADHD how they can act will frustrate them even more and contribute to a lack of faith in their ability to learn the skills they need.

Keep in mind the particular challenges of girls with ADHD: While all children with ADHD may find that their symptoms prevent them from engaging in healthy social relationships, girls with ADHD may encounter societal stereotypes of how they should act. They might be thought weird, socially distractible, too brusque, bossy, or possess other characteristics that society, including many infants, parents, and teachers, are not taught to value in girls.

Take advantage of ADHD's benefits and energy: While ADHD does have its drawbacks, it can also have a tremendous sense of imagination, high energy, and, in some cases, considerable charm. For parents, the old adage "feed the starving bee" is a good mantra. Find out what your kid enjoys doing and inspire them to continue doing it. Let's presume your child enjoys working with equipment or disassembling objects. Maybe get them a construction kit to see if they want to help you repair stuff around the home. To put it another way, figure out what hobbies and tasks they like (or at least tolerate), and let them know if there's something they just don't want to do. Who knows, if your child is given the opportunity, he or she may discover a talent for folding laundry or enjoy the responsibility of ironing shirts!

Recognize and channel children's interests: As previously mentioned, many children with ADHD may create specialized areas of interest. For example, they may struggle to finish their homework, but athletics, drama, or robotics may inspire them. You should assist your child in developing skills in an environment where he or she has a strong desire, and your child would be more encouraged to gain independence and discipline in that area. If your child loves singing, for example, they can set a target of participating at a school concert, and you may assist them in developing a practice routine. This experience will teach your child the value of hard work and breaking down planning into gradual, manageable steps over time. When it comes to conventional homework, your child will be more likely to internalize these lessons.

Take personal time to recuperate: Parents with children with ADHD can feel tired, disappointed, or even lonely at times. They must have to look after themselves as well. If at all practicable, set aside time to think and unwind. You may also find it beneficial to attend a support group for parents with children with ADHD, where you can share your thoughts and solutions with other parents dealing with similar issues. Connecting with other parents who appreciate your situation may also help to alleviate any feelings of loneliness you might be experiencing.

- Communicating Effectively with Your Child

When communicating with your infant, make sure you are expressing your demands, rules, and requests in a simple and coherent manner. Patience is important here, even though it can be difficult to find at times. Since children with ADHD may not have formed an innate understanding of how they can act, they must be reminded of their responsibilities and often motivated to complete them with external motivators.

Make straightforward requests of your child, broken down into small chunks. Some parents, for example, will need to make a list of each assignment their child needs to do before getting ready for school in the morning. Other parents will need to warn their children many hours ahead of time that they will only be allowed to play until their homework is done.

Consequences must be clearly articulated since children profit from straightforward laws and instruction. Although it can be tempting to make exceptions, particularly if a child is misbehaving, disrupting the routine is often worse. These types of improvements will affect a developing sense of obligation, depending on how the child learns.

Children can need additional motivation to complete tasks before they have internalized what they need to do. These don't have to be expensive items; popcorn works well as a treat before, during, or after your child's tasks. Sitting with your child as they do homework will help them develop a sense of obligation.

Children with ADHD frequently need early warning of what they would do in order to practice. Making urgent demands on them and then being enraged because they are not met may be inefficient. Instead, consider ahead of time about the general guidelines or steps that children must obey, and then create in extra time for your child with ADHD to perform these activities.

If your kid fails to follow through with their duties, kindly inform them of the outcome and put it into action as soon as possible. Taking away a doll or shutting off the tv, for example, is an example of this. Children with ADHD must be able to see the imminent consequences of their acts, otherwise they would be unable to comprehend the consequences of their actions. Immediate effects are more effective than long-term or ambiguous consequences. Like many children with ADHD suffer from poor self-confidence and a sense of self-worth, refrain from making intimate or disrespectful remarks. Instead, the penalties for failing to complete what they are required to do should be concrete. Children with ADHD must trust that their parents would follow through on the implications they discussed in advance.

When children get older, parents may start talking to them more freely about what it means to have ADHD. They should explain what ADHD is to children in age-appropriate terms and make it clear that they have a disorder that allows them to learn ways to deal with and with it. ADHD should not be seen as a flaw or a mistake, but rather as a characteristic of their academic style and how they interact with the environment, which allows them to be more creative and work harder in certain respects than their peers. Medical practitioners like psychiatrists and educators will also help children understand what it is to have ADHD and how it affects their lives and coping styles.

• Helping Your Child Thrive

You play a critical role in assisting your ADHD kid in reaching his or her full potential. Today, medication, alternative therapies, and strategies to help children control their ADHD at home and at school are all available.

- Working with Others on a Treatment Plan

While you may try to take on the whole burden of caring for your child on your own, it is usually important to collaborate with others in order for your child to succeed. Doctors, psychiatrists, therapists, educators, behaviorists, teachers, and other experts can be part of this team at times. While working with so many people can sound daunting, each specialist has a role to play in supporting your child. You do not need any of them, but it is useful to be aware of how they can help you and your kids.

To begin, your child may be eligible for educational benefits under the Americans with Disabilities Act (ADA) and the Individuals with Disabilities Education Act (IDEA) (IDEA). You may ask for an Individualized Education Program (IEP), which is a specialized, personalized education package geared to your child's needs. In an ideal future, any school will have a fantastic special education curriculum, but you will need to lobby for your child's needs to the school administrators.

An IEP considers a child's talents as well as the fact that the child has clear learning and growth goals, which are then identified. There should be processes in place to assess if such needs are being fulfilled. Your child may also be entitled to special considerations, such as more time on standardized exams or the use of audiobooks or other assistive technology. For further details, contact the Department of Education.

It's important to communicate with the people who deal with your child on a daily basis, and to be transparent and truthful with them. For example, you should report the habits you see your child display at home as accurately as possible. Medication dosages, recovery schedules, and learning objectives can need to be updated in certain situations. Checking in with your child's staff on a regular basis is therefore important to ensure that their therapies are current. Be sure the child's doctor is aware of any side effects you're experiencing since some of them can be dangerous. If you wish to stop taking a treatment or drug, rather than working on your own, remind your staff. Medications must normally be tapered off with the help of a doctor. You may also encourage your child to keep an age-appropriate journal of their observations of the treatments, which can help them develop independence while also offering useful knowledge.

Receiving and implementing input from too many different sources can be overwhelming at times. Request advice from friends or school personnel for practitioners who have successfully assisted other children with ADHD. Whether you like you can't talk freely with someone on your child's support staff, or if they're pushing a treatment that doesn't appear to be working, try to find someone with whom you can work more cooperatively. This isn't to say that the other one will necessarily say what you want to hear, but there are a variety of recovery options available. Physicians, clinicians, and learning counsellors should still be willing to tailor their therapies to the child's unique requirements. There is no such thing as a one-size-fits-all solution. Ensure that the staff has time to meet with you outside of your child's meetings to ensure that they are receiving the most complete information from you and that you are getting the most complete information from them.

- Medication

Only a qualified doctor will assist you in selecting a prescription for your infant. Your doctor may have prior experience dealing with children who have ADHD. If your child has some of the above-mentioned coexisting illnesses, the doctor should be familiar with treating them as well. This segment will introduce you to several popular drugs used to treat ADHD in children, as well as their side effects, although it is not meant to substitute professional medical recommendations on the best treatment for your child.

Some medicines operate right away, while others take a while to produce results. Furthermore, the drug can have the opposite effect on your infant at first, making them become more agitated before their bodies respond to it. While the quest for the best prescription for your child may be stressful, bear in mind that psychiatry for children normally entails some trial and error, not only with the dose, but also with various prescriptions or combinations of medications. Share any side effects you notice with your child's doctor during this phase. Keep a diary of your child's thoughts or behavior, and ask your child to do the same at an age-appropriate stage, as previously described.

Your staff should be checking up on you and your child on a daily basis, since a doctor should not only administer drugs without having a structure of follow-up appointments. Furthermore, the doctor will choose to give you and your child's teachers paperwork to fill out that ask about your child's symptoms; this material can be used to determine the treatment's effectiveness.

Amphetamine

Amphetamine is thought to act as an ADHD treatment by rising dopamine levels in the brain. People with ADHD normally have lower levels of this neurotransmitter, and the dopamine levels by stimulant therapy can help to relax and concentrate their minds. Adderall (mixed amphetamine salts) and Dexedrine are the two most common amphetamines used for ADHD (dextroamphetamine). They're mostly administered as short-acting pills that run for four to six hours, but some kids will need to take another dose or half of a dose later in the day.

Adderall XR, Dexedrine XR, and Vyvanse XR are some of the longer-acting (extended-release, or XR) forms of these drugs that last eight to twelve hours (lisdexamfetamine). Loss of appetite, weight loss, sleep loss, tics, frustration, and irritable behavior are some of the side effects associated with this type of drugs. These side effects, however, do not exist with all children who take these medications. After being familiar with the medicine's influence, some children and adults may find it easier to take non-time-release tablets.

Methylphenidate Stimulants

Methylphenidate, a central nervous system stimulant, is present in this family of drugs, which includes Focalin and Ritalin. Many are short films, running four to six hours, but there are also extended-release versions available. Medication with a shorter half-life can need additional doses during the day. Appetite loss, insomnia, weight loss, irritability, and tics are all side effects of this class of drugs. Such medicines, such as the Daytrana patch, distribute drugs directly to the bloodstream via the scalp, bypassing the digestive system. This kind of patch eliminates the need for children to swallow tablets or contact their school nurses for afternoon doses. The patch can cause skin irritation and have similar side effects to other methylphenidate stimulants.

Nonstimulants are substances that do not stimulate the central nervous system.

Amphetamines are not present in this class of drugs. Strattera (atomoxetine) improves concentration, working memory, and impulse control while decreasing distractibility by rising norepinephrine, which controls attention and thereby reduces impulsivity and hyperactivity, and Intuniv (guanfacine), which acts on brain receptors to enhance attention, working memory, and impulse control while decreasing distractibility. Insomnia, nausea, agitation, sore stomach, dizziness, dry mouth, and, in rare cases, liver damage are all common Strattera side effects. Strattera has been linked to an uptick in suicidal ideation. Sleepiness, nausea, headaches, stomach pain, and, in rare cases, decreased blood pressure and variations in heart rate can also be side effects of Intuniv.

Antidepressants

Antidepressants like Wellbutrin (bupropion) come in fast- and long-acting versions, and they're often offered to kids with ADHD. Wellbutrin can cause sleep disturbances, headaches, and, in extreme cases, seizures. Antidepressants are often given to infants who cannot tolerate stimulant drugs or who have tics or insomnia. Antidepressants help to relieve signs of inattention, impulsivity, and hyperactivity.

Blood Pressure Medications

Children with ADHD are often offered blood pressure drugs, such as clonidine. Clonidine should be used alone or in conjunction with stimulant medicine to help with ADHD symptoms. It can also help with anger and insomnia from stimulant medication. Clonidine can make you feel tired, dizzy, irritable, have low blood pressure, and have a dry mouth.

Although treatment may help children cope with the effects of ADHD, it does not cure the condition. Instead, the right drug at the right dosage will help a child stay calm, mitigate hyperactivity, and curb impulsivity so that they can concentrate on daily activities and follow techniques that can help them be more active. To put it another way, drugs work well when they're paired with educational and social therapies aimed at helping a child develop positive planning, organizing, and learning techniques.

- **Alternative Therapies**

Alternative therapies have helped certain children with ADHD, and your child can learn from them as well. It's just a case of putting them to the test to see what works. While there is a general lack of scientific research behind these forms of therapy, anecdotal evidence suggests that many of these methods are effective. Allow enough time for the benefits to kick in, as for most treatment. When you deal with a pro in these areas, they will be able to tell you how long you will have to wait for results.

✓ Modified Diets

Although sugar has long been blamed for causing ADHD, there is no scientific evidence to support this argument. Sugar and refined carbohydrates, such as white flour goods, will, on the other hand, raise a child's activity level by releasing sugar into the bloodstream. Furthermore, many people with ADHD (both adults and children) self-medicate with sugary foods, and whether you or your child has this problem, it's best to break it as soon as possible. Especially if they are on medication to control their hyperactivity, the dopamine surge caused by a sugar rush will lead children to become more hyperactive. A healthy diet will help all children, not just those with ADHD, maintain their blood glucose levels during the day. Children's overall health benefits from a diet rich in fruits, vegetables, and whole grain products like oatmeal and whole wheat bread.

Any parents have had success with their children following the Feingold diet, which was created by allergist Benjamin Feingold, MD. To prevent hyperactivity, he recommends avoiding foods that contain artificial dyes, flavorings, or preservatives. Although scientific evidence for the Feingold diet is lacking, some parents say it has helped their children become less hyperactive.

Children with ADHD can have a low level of omega-3 fatty acids in their blood, according to research, and may benefit from supplements. Children with ADHD demonstrated a slight but significant reduction of symptoms in randomized trials with an intervention and placebo sample.

An elimination diet is often used by parents to rule out foods that may aggravate their children's ADHD symptoms. This diet will recognize potential culprits that cause a children's behavior by removing or adding those forms of food at specific times and measuring the results. If you want to pursue an elimination diet for your child, consult with a doctor and a nutritionist to guarantee that your child continues to eat a well-balanced diet throughout the process.

✓ Cognitive Behavioral Therapy for ADHD

While cognitive behavioral therapy (CBT) was originally designed to help people deal with depression and anxiety, it may also help people with ADHD learn to alter the thoughts and behaviors that exacerbate their ADHD symptoms and contribute to disorganization and bad time management. CBT patients also collaborate in groups with a consultant to work on topics including organizational and time management skills. When opposed to conventional supportive therapy, participants in these community services saw results. These services are more effective for older, more verbal children and adults. Individualized CBT counselling sessions are also available.

✓ Neurofeedback

Any people with ADHD have had experience with neurofeedback therapy. This biofeedback technique helps a person to track their own brain function using sensors on their head that relay audio or visual signals to a computer. Patients will gradually learn to control their own brain function as they gain this awareness. However, many people agree that further research is needed to assess the feasibility of this form of ADHD training. Also, keep in mind that neurofeedback can be costly and time-consuming.

- ✓ Working Memory Training (COGMED)

Any individuals with ADHD have problems with working memory, which can make it difficult to perform memory-related tasks. Working memory is the short-term memory that retains and preserves incoming information; it is the capacity to keep information in the mind for a short amount of time and use it before it is passed to long-term memory. Working memory is critical for learning and conceptual manipulation of symbols, as well as other cognitive tasks. COGMED training involves using a computer programme to improve attention and problem-solving capabilities while also increasing working memory capability and capacity. While studies have shown some short-term changes in working memory, the findings so far indicate that only visual memory is improved over time with this form of therapy.

- ✓ Meditation

Some people with ADHD can depend on the adrenaline rush that comes with being overly stimulated to motivate them to take action. They can, for example, be able to focus on projects only when they can no longer procrastinate, triggering a stress response that prompts them to act. This constant flood of adrenaline, on the other hand, has a negative impact on both the body and the mind. Anyone may be harmed by it, and their immunity can be reduced as a result.

An individual with ADHD can benefit from meditation to relax their body and mind to counteract this. While it can be difficult to teach children, especially younger ones, to sit in silence, anybody may learn basic strategies over time, such as repeating a mantra with their eyes closed or focusing on their breath intake or exhalation. To help them concentrate their mind and vision, they can need a focal object, such as a toy or beloved stuffed animal.

If you think meditation might help your child, try it with them and ask them what sounds most calming and soothing to them. Specific visualization techniques, in which children go on an imaginary, relaxing adventure, can also help very imaginative children.

If a child is unable to stay still, they will be able to meditate more effectively by doing yoga or moderate exercise such as walking. They might enjoy meditating outdoors in a tranquil setting, such as by the ocean or a lake, or in a wooded clearing. They can begin by focusing and calming their minds by paying attention to the sensory stimuli around them, such as bird calls or waves.

- ✓ Equine Therapy

Equine-assisted psychotherapy helps some children with ADHD. This method of rehabilitation involves incorporating horses into a treatment programme aimed at assisting an individual in achieving specific objectives. The infant understands the horse's moods and discovers the horse's desires when learning to ride a horse, becoming less dependent on themselves and more able to understand how their actions effect others.

To increase self-awareness, equine-assisted psychotherapy normally includes debriefing with a psychologist during one's interaction with the horse. Children's effects of inattention, hyperactivity, and impulsivity may be reduced by engaging with horses and observing how their behavior influences them, according to several reports.

Horses are also well-liked by children because they respond without judgement or criticism and make their needs evident. When combined with this immediate and visible guidance lesson, children can gain trust in their ability to guide a powerful animal like a horse. Anxiety and depression have also been found to be reduced with this type of therapy.

Modifying Your Parenting Approach

QUIZ: WHAT ARE YOUR CHILD'S ADHD CHALLENGES?

This quiz will help you pinpoint your child's unique problems and refine your understanding of the kinds of concerns they're dealing with so you can come up with the best ways to help them. Check the habits that matter to your child depending on how much they occur, and use this information to help your child develop a recovery plan.

1. *My child is often restless.*
2. *My child daydreams constantly.*
3. *My child is angry or explosive.*
4. *My child loses belongings.*
5. *My child is prone to injury.*
6. *My child loses track of time.*
7. *My child speaks out of turn.*
8. *My child cannot keep up with conversations.*
9. *My child struggles with insomnia.*
10. *My child is always lagging behind others.*

Your child could be dealing with impulsivity and hyperactivity if you replied "yes" or "sometimes" to several of the odd-numbered statements. Ways to relax your child's mind and harness their energies productively should be included in the strategy you build for them. You'll need to schedule time for your kid to be physically involved. Be honest about how much focus your child will provide during more sedentary or boring tasks. Your child might be very inventive with boundless energy to try new things.

If you replied "yes" or "sometimes" to the even-numbered statements the majority of the time, your child could be dealing with inattention. Your strategy would be to assist your child in attending school and keeping track of hours, possessions, and other tasks. It's possible that your child may need to schedule peaceful everyday events that don't confuse them. Your child could be a creative person who daydreams and creates art, stories, or other inventions during periods of inattention.

If you answered "yes" or "sometimes" to both the odd and even questions, your child might be suffering from inattention, hyperactivity, or impulsivity. In this situation, the strategy should focus on ways to help the child focus while still reducing or channeling hyperactivity and impulsivity. Your child can be a creative individual with a lot of enthusiasm and the ability to turn their imaginative ideas into reality.

NOTE: The purpose of this quiz is to help you identify some

of your child's habits that you'd like to fix and improve. It is not meant to be diagnostic or to take the place of a doctor's or psychologist's assessment. If you need more details, ask your psychiatrist or counsellor to go through your child's condition with you in greater depth. If your child was tested by a psychologist, the psychoeducational assessment provided by the counsellor will provide you with very nuanced and accurate knowledge on how your child's mind functions. If you're having trouble understanding the assessment, schedule a meeting with the counsellor to read through the results and have the psychologist explain the conclusions in layman's terms.

You should adapt your parenting approach to take into account your child's talents, challenges, desires, priorities, and opportunities based on the results of the questionnaire and what you know about your child. Here's how to do it:

First, evaluate your child's vast talents and remind yourself of all the wonderful characteristics he or she possesses. For eg, your child could be artistic, perceptive to others, courageous, athletic, or any number of other qualities. You should apply these characteristics to your parenting style. When your kid is perceptive, they will use their imagination to study other people's coping mechanisms to see if they work with them.

Second, evaluate the child's difficulties and areas of improvement. For example, your child may be inattentive, have difficulties doing assignments, and/or initiating tasks; they may also struggle to get along with peers, resulting in moodiness.

Third, based on your child's talents and challenges, create any concrete expectations that you and your child will work toward in the coming months. It may be feasible for your child to keep a homework log in a diary, on a tablet, or on another unit. Simply write the start time of each project and how long it took to finish the job to help them stay on track. This will assist you and your child in developing a series of targets that are both attainable and observable. If your child is outgoing, they may like to join an after-school study group to help them get started on their homework.

Finally, think about the tools you'll need to help your girl. If your kid is concerned about the social stresses of attending a homework group, they will be able to focus on peer relations with the school psychologist or therapists (or other members of your team of helpers). Resources may include area service centers and associations, religious or other organizations, and ADHD support groups, in addition to the school and the ADHD support team.

• Sample Parenting Approaches

Different children can necessitate a variety of parenting styles. Consider Emily, a timid, inattentive ten-year-old with demonstrable abilities. Emily is a gifted and dedicated reader as well as a compassionate soul who is still composing poetry. Her difficulties stem from her distractibility, which causes her to abandon assignments or fail to complete them. She always misplaces her purse, scarves, and homework, and she struggles to make friends and keep up with her classmates. She enjoys contributing in class, but she has a tendency to make statements that are unrelated to other students' comments, prompting other students to laugh at her. She is easily irritated by critique. Even gentle advice from her parents and teachers will elicit intense reactions or tears.

Emily's practical approach entails frequent oral and written updates about what she has to do to stay on track. It will be critical to keep her engaged and inspired by using her interests and talents (in this case, her poetry). She might, for example, compose a poem to remind herself of what she wants to get done every day or do a ten-minute free write before starting her homework to help her concentrate. Emily's parents should make a point of praising her accomplishments on a daily basis and redirecting her when she makes a mistake rather than criticizing or shouting. Emily will attend intramural clubs at school and make friends with other students who love writing or theatre if she so desires.

To make the most of the opportunities available to their daughter, Emily's parents should schedule appointments with her teachers to discuss Emily's interests and to let them know that she wishes to participate in class discussions but doesn't really know how. This strategy can also be implemented with the assistance of the school's special education department, which often serves as a link between parents and teachers.

Remember Jake, a rambunctious nine-year-old who loves swimming and video games. He is a witty young man who enjoys doing stand-up comedy routines and excels in athletics. He is normally unable to obey instructions at home or at school, and he is irritable and vulnerable to injury. In training, he fidgets a lot, and tasks that demand constant concentration frustrate him. Jake has trouble controlling his emotions and can become irritable. He is prone to violent outbursts in response to criticism, and he often clashes with his siblings.

Jake's creativity can be channeled and used as a parental strategy. Swimming is a discipline that does not require relentless guidance and has a low chance of injury, so he should be allowed to keep swimming. If Jake is excited, he could go for a morning swim at the nearby community center before school to clear his head and burn off some steam. After he has been busy, he will need to attend to homework and activities that require more focus, otherwise he will not be able to finish them. Clear and consistent instructions should be given to him. If he becomes enraged when he is criticized, he needs to be offered a quiet place to calm down apart from his siblings. His parents should react to his outbursts as politely as possible, as their indignation would only exacerbate his behavior. Jake's parents should make a list of things that he has to do each afternoon and reward him with time spent playing video games if he completes them and sticks to it. They may even set up a basketball hoop in the basement for him and enroll him in morning swim at the nearby community center.

You may find it useful to break down your parenting strategy like this:

1. Your child's strengths

2. Your child's challenges

3. Realistic goals for you and your child to achieve in a reasonable amount of time

4. The resources needed to accomplish these goals

For example, here's how the parents of a nine-year-old

fourth grader named

For instance, consider how the parents of a nine-year-old fourth-grader named Sydney might break down their parenting approach:

- Strengths: She is energetic, inventive, and enjoys playing music.

- Challenges: She may be impulsive, talk out of order, and erupt into rages because she believes others do not understand her. Furthermore, despite her intelligence, she has difficulty understanding the steps in math equations and reading comprehension.

Sydney will begin partnering with the after-school tutoring service at school in the coming month, concentrating on math and literacy. She will begin working with a girls' ADHD support group in the next two months. Each instructor will award her with a star for each day she does not interrupt, fight with peers, or get out of her seat, using a star system. She will collect and exchange these stars for breaks, such as playing music at recess.

Sydney would need to sign up for Sydney's school's after-school study hours. Her parents will inquire about the timetable for the girls' programme at a nearby ADHD support group. Sydney's teacher will create a behavior chart that will monitor her academic progress.

• The Supportive Family

Although you may be excited to pursue a new parenting method for your kids, bear in mind that making improvements often requires both victories and failures. Enlist the help of the child's siblings, relatives, and caregivers to incorporate the new strategy so that the child receives clear responses and discipline from all.

Make sure your expectations for yourself, your child, and the rest of your family are reasonable. Although any parent wishes the best for their child and their family as a whole, it's important to remember that long-term progress takes time. You, your child, and the rest of the family will remain encouraged if your aspirations are achievable, measurable, and evolving. Instead of setting ambitious expectations where you would lose momentum before seeing them realized, plan for the next few months.

Getting your other children to comply with your efforts to support your child with ADHD can be complicated at times. They may be resentful of their sibling receiving what they consider to be more recognition from you and others.

In this situation, make sure to provide incentives and recognition for their contributions in order to help the ADHD parenting strategy. Often, keep in mind that children sometimes become accustomed to playing specific roles in the family. While the child tries to improve their attitudes and position in the family, the other children will respond negatively or resentfully toward their ADHD sibling.

You will combat this by simply expressing to the whole family that, regardless of any modifications that occur, everyone in the family has a special place. Small victories in the road to progress should be rewarded and celebrated as a family. The path may be bumpy and slow, but you will arrive on the other side!

CHAPTER 5
Teaching Your Child Self-Care

Our first goal is to help your child develop his or her self-care. You will, of course, get assistance if necessary, but it will be better to her if she is able to administer her self-care individually. Since she would be more able to follow along if she is excited to be self-sufficient, the tactics in this chapter are designed to encourage her excitement.

Rather than relying on your verbal instructions, it is preferable if your child learns to perform self-care in response to signals in her environment when acquiring autonomy. Teach her to use an alarm clock instead of your voice to get up. Often think about your daughter as a success: imagine her learning to brush her own teeth, pour her own glass of milk, wear a watch, pick her own shoes, and dress herself. And very young children can do these tasks, and you can expect the same for your boy.

It's possible that your child lacks an age-appropriate sense of responsibility. According to a report, children with ADHD lag behind their peers by 30% when it comes to self-management skills. Until you order your kid to wash her hands after using the restroom, clean up after herself, brush her teeth, unzip her jacket, and so on, she is unable to do so. So why is it that she is unaware of these simple customs and rituals?

- Emphasizing the Advantages

If you attempt to teach self-care to your girl, she will react negatively to your efforts. She may feel as though you're walking away from her, pressuring her to do more work and robbing her of your time and companionship. When this occurs, she may be avoiding the most critical task at hand: self-care.

Parental efforts to support their children's self-care, similar to weaning, are driving more children away. Children are unable to give up the love that comes from their families, but they fear being rejected because their parents are not involved in any aspect of their lives. They may be concerned that any self-sustaining actions, especially that of their siblings, would cause their parents to focus on other matters.

If you believe this is the case, ask your child the rhetorical question, "Do you think I'd forget about you if you take better care of yourself?" 'I'm wondering if you'd like to spend some time growing up with me,' and imagine what you might do together.

Assist your child in comprehending the benefits of self-reliance. For example, without you, she will be able to go more places, people will be less critical of her, and she will be able to complete projects while no one else is available. You want her to understand that by practicing good self-care, she can gain more than she losses. The language you use and the sound of your voice will have an impact on which she responds favorably, and it's still a good idea to keep track of her self-care progress and ability to support others.

Helping Your Child Follow Through Independently

It's important to assist your daughter in doing what she said she'll do without having to prompt her. Scientists have devised a method to assist citizens in carrying out their plans. If you assist your child with "planning for success" in this manner, there is a greater risk that she can carry out her plan immediately on her own.

As if you were rehearsing for a play, ask your child to tell you what she's going to do and why, where, and how she'll do it. Then teach her to know the cues that will prompt her to carry out her plan in the area. You should take a step back and let her be guided by the setting. She is supposed to be more determined to step through now that she has taken the lead.

This strategy may have amazing results. For example, if your daughter needs to remember to return a library book at the end of the week, she will place the book next to her musical instrument, which she usually brings to school for Friday group practice. This will encourage her to see the book before she leaves the house on that particular day, indicating her return.

- POOR HYGIENE

You can keep telling your child to brush or shower, but this isn't always the right answer. Often, if your child is reliant on your efforts, she will not learn to cope on her own. She'll also be annoyed by your daily reminders and think you doubt her performance.

Since your child is aware that you are concerned with her appearance, failure to fulfil your demands might become an effective tactic used to intimidate you when she is angry. Furthermore, if she enjoys the fact that you are concerned about her, she will be unable to give up. When children overreact to hygiene issues, they are always advised that their parents are concerned about them. There may be a variety of explanations for a child's inability to follow basic self-care routines. Here are a few examples.

- Robert was affected by poor modeling; his parents preserved their grooming by copying the mediocre style.

- Fine motor problems clashed with Michael's self-care; he suffered more than others did, and his parents got accustomed to taking control of themselves.

- Philip felt safer when his body smell kept others at the length of his arm.

Identifying what is hampering the child in this field is important. Fortunately, children do not always see sanitation in a negative light. For starters, when they get in, kids are often hesitant to get out of the shower. An inability to begin a hygiene-related project seems to have very little to do with the negative operation.

- Solutions

Negative words and coercion may have a negative impact on your child's hygiene reaction, which is often a factor in resistance. Checking to see whether she washed her hands with soap, or requesting that she do so, would just make hand washing a chore she dislikes. If you're having a hard time washing your hands, you might ask her: "What really is going on? Are you okay with letting germs live on your paws, or are you irritated when you feel like I'm running you around?" Maintaining a good attitude, maintaining satisfaction, and complimenting your child's abilities will help her to keep her room clean.

Let's take a look at tooth brushing as an example. You should ask your daughter whether she needs to take care of her teeth and when she wants to brush them. You might say, "When she has a recommendation," if she has one "The dentist recommends cleaning them for each meal. This makes the teeth healthy and strong.

Prevent your child from being dependent on you. Rather than cleaning the child's teeth, show her how to do it. "I will show you how the dentist taught me," you can say. Assist her in recognizing that she takes excellent care of herself while she manages her grooming. Healthy teeth need less maintenance work (which is never fun), and your child will appreciate it if people see her beautiful smile and compliment her on it.

However, your child may be checking whether or not she has the right to refuse a request for hygiene, and you should consider this rather than insist on it.

The world will not stop if her life deteriorates for a brief period of time. Your child's immune system can be weakened if you don't exert pressure all of the time. "Choose your battles," as the saying goes. Your child's inadequate grooming can have nothing to do with their inability to comprehend the consequences of their actions. As you might be aware, often people torture themselves in order to make a point.

If the issue continues, a fact check might be necessary. You want your daughter to understand the consequences of being irresponsible. It was crucial to remind Nick that if he forgot to use his orthodontic "appliance," for example, his error could result in serious jaw malformation. "Isn't it much worth wearing to you?" the mother asked. When your back is to the wall, you should always ask yourself, "Would you be able to do that if you didn't want to?" After all, most of us do things we don't want to do. Conscientious self-care, like most highly appropriate practices, conscientious self-care requires commitment to plans and other constraints whether we like it or not. We've both seen this inconvenience, and even though we aren't completely oblivious to it, we realize that we must comply. Assume your child is capable of doing the same.

• Developing Routines

Establishing everyday rituals for activities like washing your hands and body and brushing your teeth is important. That is how the majority of people's welfare is guaranteed. Help your child recognize environmental cues that will prompt her to brush and wash her teeth. For example, the invitation to begin a meal may indicate that she had washed her hands.

Putting on her pajamas will serve as a cue to brush her teeth. The aim, as always, is to create a schedule that she can follow without you.

Instead of spelling out each step, you might say, "It's getting late" or "We've got to leave fast" if your daughter doesn't follow her schedule. Rather than asking her what to do, this would give her a better chance to control herself. "Is there anything else you'd like to do before you go to sleep?" you might ask if you notice she skipped a phase in her bedtime routine, such as brushing her teeth. As a last resort, you can ask "Are you sure you don't want to brush your teeth before going to bed?"

• Being Firm

Forcing a child to do grooming makes no sense because there is no other option, and this will only succeed if she is very young and easily overwhelmed physically. However, setting firm boundaries will strengthen your child's desire to obey. "We might need to use some of our film money to pay the dentist for extra appointments," you may suggest if she continues to ignore her teeth. "You may prefer not to scrub, but in that case, it's better better not to buy the goodies that might be harmful for your teeth," you might add if her lack of self-care also leaves her susceptible to cavities. You don't want to inflict pain on your child; instead, you protect her and don't harm her. Whether or not it bothers her, you're determined to solve a dilemma and take decisive action. The technique teaches her that her loss affects others as much as herself.

• Ostracizing

In certain serious cases, ostracizing your daughter might be sufficient to resolve her lack of grooming. "We'd love to have you join us, but only if you're willing to shower and get ready in clean clothes," you might say, because it's important to be considerate to others. If she continues to refuse, you might want to ask her, "Is there any excuse to cause such a family conflict? Were you preoccupied with anything else?" If things don't change, unless you can find someone to live with her at home when you're gone, you may have to leave your child behind. We should consider the financial burden on the family if you have to pay someone to keep an eye on her. You should let her pay the sitter with her own cash (or sell any of her toys if she doesn't have any). Well, she has the ability to sabotage, but she still misses the trip and contributes personal funds to compensate for the inconvenience. She then determines whether or not sanitation should be ignored.

• DIFFICULTIES WITH DRESS

Since your child is going to struggle with folding, buttoning, and zipping, it's important that she learns these skills. Unfortunately, she will not be happy about giving up your assistance. "Ma!" she might exclaim, for example. Then casually raise her leg and wait for you to place her sock on it. If you don't help her, you might feel guilty, but you're not perpetuating laziness or dominance by doing so.

Alternatively, only have enough assistance to enable you to progress slowly. If you don't help your daughter as soon as she tears or says, "I can't," her self-care skills will deteriorate. Inviting her to clarify why she is reluctant to do anything is a positive first step toward keeping the ball in her possession.

• Solutions

Helping your child learn self-help skills takes time. You won't have the option of waiting for her to fix and develop challenges if you're rushed and under pressure to get things finished. She will be disturbed and disappointed if she doubts her ability and learn and fulfil standards quickly enough. This problem can be avoided if you plan ahead of time, then things can run more smoothly. To begin, explore clothing choices the night before, while you have time to work together. It's preferable to being frantic in the morning when time is limited.

If your child has greater control of her clothing, she will likely have more confidence and cooperation. Instead of asking her what to wear on a chilly day, you might just say, "It's cold outside." This would give her the impression that she has more influence of her wardrobe choices. When she grows older, she may be able to check the weather on her own.

• Clothing Decisions

You may need to rely on those clothing to shield your child from the elements or to ensure that her wardrobe is appropriate. However, her clothing selections are frequently not enough provocative to warrant punitive action. Your daughter will not catch a cold because she is underdressed, as your child's pediatrician will tell you; she will just be cold. And if she gets cold enough, she'll actually make different decisions in the future. Natural causes have that kind of power.

You may be concerned that if your daughter does not wear such clothing, a family outing will be ruined. You may be concerned that if you can't go back, she may become depressed and cause problems for others. In these situations, you might tell her to carry a few extra items "just in case." It may also be beneficial to find a safe way to transport the extra clothing (so that she does not feel burdened). Instead of demanding a solution, choose one that is suitable for all of you.

Make sure she knows when your daughter has to dress a certain way. Consider the following example: "These are the sorts of outfits we put on for church. Which one do you want to put on today?" There are moments where you have very few options. When your kid starts to cry, there may be other explanations for her refusal to cooperate. It's not always a matter of clothing, just as it's not always a matter of hygiene, so see if she's bothered by anything else. That should suffice to solve the issue.

However, just when you say anything to your daughter doesn't mean she gets her way. To begin, if you bring home clothes you've purchased for her and she refuses to wear them, let her say, "I can wait until tomorrow, but then I'll have to return them to the shop." This kind of mundane outcome could pique her interest and encourage her to try on the new clothes sooner. If you're always having issues with clothes for her, look for them just when she's around.

• Wearing the same outfit

It can make you uncomfortable if your child continues to wear the same outfit for many days in a row. You may be concerned that allowing this to happen would make you reckless, as well as concerned about her grubby appearance and how some will react.

When you're worried about your daughter's connection to

her wardrobe, consider this: if she looks disheveled, is it really that bad? Is it really worth arguing about? If she says yes, you might say to her: "I know you're a fan of the pants and top. I'll see how I can wash the shirt and make it last longer. After the top is dry, I'll wash the trousers for you." With this approach, your daughter keeps half of the outfit throughout the cleaning process.

You may believe that your child will continue to wear filthy clothes.

• DIFFICULTIES WITH SLEEP

Since sleep is so important for your child's health, it's critical to maintain a healthy sleep routine. Getting up early every morning (with no naps during the day) will assist your child in establishing a healthy 24-hour cycle known as a circadian rhythm. Variations in weekend sleep schedules will make it difficult for your child to get up for school on Monday morning, so try to keep it consistent. If your child has healthy sleeping habits, she will naturally learn to wake up at the same time every day without the use of an alarm clock.

Sleep issues are common in children living with ADHD. They have further bouts of sleepiness during the day, and their lack of sleep exacerbates their problems with behavior and school inattention. That's why it's important to figure out what's disrupting your child's sleep.

It's important to identify and address any problems that are interfering with your child's sleep. A child always resists sleep, much as she does all of the other restraints you impose. "You have to sleep," you say, and she asks, "Why?" And he comes up with an excuse to say no. It's often just a ruse to get you to speak with her. You have to abandon what you're doing, create a drama, and be worried about her well-being because she doesn't follow the bedtime schedule.

• Solutions

When you read Richard Ferber's sleep therapy, you'll understand how important it is for your child to learn to sleep without relying on you. The technique you'll find in this book is, in many ways, an expansion of the Ferber process for many of your child's issues. You are showing your kid how to manage life without your constant guidance and motivation.

The first step is to establish a schedule for your child to follow from beginning to end. From the onset, try to establish a consistent time for beginning the bedtime routine. You want her to put down her other tasks, do her laundry, and change into her pajamas so you can relax, listen, and tell stories.

You can have a reminder at first, but couple it with other

signals as soon as possible (a clock, a TV show completion, etc.). "Let's get ready for stories as soon as your show is done," you might suggest, but the point is that you want your child to respond to cues without your interference. If your daughter refuses to follow the routine you've developed, tell her you're ready to begin bedtime activities and wait for her to do so. Mention if you'll get more time together if she dies. It demonstrates that you want to share the special time set aside for you.

• Maintain Limits

You want your child to understand that bedtime has a firm start and finish while demonstrating commitment to tackle all challenges and being versatile when situations are extenuating. When the clock strikes an hour, your child will know you're out. You and your child would have less time together if you start late. If your daughter utterly disregards the bedtime routine, you will have to force her into her sleep. Setting strict boundaries would aid her in developing punctuality.

When your child emerges from her room after bedtime, do not look after her. It's also not a good idea to torture her for anything else, like taking away her tv or forcing her to go to bed earlier. Without speaking to her bed, clearly guide her. "What can we do to make your bedtime easier to end?" you can still remind her later. "How are you going to finish your bedtime?" he asks. Assist in the resolution of the issue.

• Explore obstacles

It can be daunting to establish a perfect bedtime routine; a variety of problems can arise. Mostly, one parent is disengaged, and the non-participating parent is the one who gets the fight off the couch before bedtime. Under these situations, it's important to figure out what's behind the parent's failure to participate.

• Older Children

As your child gets older, she'll also want more feedback on her bedtime routine. More problem-solving would be needed. You want her to get plenty of sleep without feeling compelled to do so. Having enough downtime to fulfil obligations to retain health and finish what she wants to do is often a challenge. "How much sleep do you want to get in the morning to feel good?" you might ask. "Is it worth losing a night's sleep to read the chapter?" he asked.

Instead of encouraging your child to stay up late to watch TV, it could be best if you record the show for her to watch later. You could also allow her to finish her schoolwork early so she has more time to enjoy herself later in the evening while other family members are around. Have an overnight routine for the rest of the family that allows them to have personal time and positive resources. However, make sure you have some versatility during this period, or negative publicity can increase.

• Difficulty Caring for Personal Belongings

If your kid expects you to clean up after her, she will not treat her personal belongings with the dignity they deserve. She can toss toys to the side without regard for the mess they create as soon as they irritate her, leaving a trail of her belongings across the house. You don't want to be her personal servant for the rest of your life, so it's critical that you take responsibility for her belongings from your child.

• Solutions

When you look at people who keep things calm and dry, you'll find three things they do on a daily basis. They wipe up the mess first, until it becomes unmanageable. Second, after they're through with an operation, they tidy up so that the space can be used for something else. Third, they return items to their assigned positions when they are no longer needed. It denotes that the items are safe and easy to find. Staying ordered isn't rocket science. It is only a matter of time before these procedures are finished.

When she teaches your daughter to think for her

possessions, help her get into the habit of cleaning up before the mess becomes intolerable and before beginning something different. You should take it easy now that you know when to cut something out. "These stuff were put away when you played the game," she might think. "Please come to the kitchen and grab your things," say if she's alone in the kitchen with her toys.

• Promoting Self-Management

If your daughter is going to take care of her own possessions, she will forego the benefit of having someone else set them up for her. She'll have to forego the benefit of seeing people scurrying around looking for anything she can't find. And she needs to work out what to do when she ends an operation that isn't yet done. We've always felt this way at some point: throwing things aside when there's a legitimate excuse to keep them handy isn't really worth it.

Many that want things to be extremely smooth and tidy have a tendency to set things down, even though they might need them again in the future. They don't mind the additional work because they despise clutter and are extremely defensive of their belongings. Your boy, on the other hand, may opt for the opposite. She will put an end to the hard work, deal with the confusion, and seize the moment when items go missing or are hurt. As is apparent in almost every facet of life, each side has its benefits, and the middle ground usually has the fewest drawbacks.

The value of preserving a certain object, the cleaning challenge, and the implications of coping with the mess can all influence an individual's organisational behavior. A disorganized bedroom or playroom, for example, has more ramifications than the same untidiness in the middle of the kitchen floor. All of this can be confusing, but it just ensures that the child may need to develop various habits depending on the situation.

• Set firm limits

I can assure you that if your daughter gets so much, she will be irresponsible about her belongings. She would be less able to protect her belongings if you replace them too soon. She won't have any problem with the mess she leaves if you clean up after her. While some children are too tired or distressed to expend their energies to spend time with their personal possessions to be attentive, many children want their parents to tidy up after them. They still believe that their parents can find or repair any missing things. Carelessness is sometimes allowed to continue due to disciplinary incompetence.

So, if you feel like your child is treating you like a maid or butler, stand straight and steady. "I love you a lot, and I'm just a little sad, but I keep seeing candy wrappers all over the house," tell if she doesn't pick up her candy wrappers. Request her assistance in resolving the problem, but if that fails, say, "I don't know what else to do except stop buying candy before I see you tidy up after yourself." "Let's put these stuff in storage so you'll have fewer to look at," you might suggest. We will add more toys if dealing with all of that isn't too much of a headache for you." You should also tell her that putting toys underfoot sends the message that she doesn't care for them. "If you don't have a better plan, I'll hide the toys and keep them out of everyone's way," she says. "They're in the attic," you might say if you end up taking this action and she objects. Since they've been sitting there for days, I assumed you didn't care about them. However, putting so much emphasis on cleaning up after yourself can lead to your child refusing to clean up a mess until it's completely cleaned up. Since she's heard you say "I'm not putting it away, I haven't taken it out," your daughter might learn to say "I'm not putting it away, I haven't taken it out." Under this scenario, one might claim that assisting others would not always inspire them to be lazy. A mistake is not always the result of incompetence, because if anyone pitches in and lends a hand, there is no drawback.

• POOR MONEY MANAGEMENT

Children and adults with ADHD have a pattern of spending

money recklessly. Their condition can deteriorate to the point that their families and spouses are forced to expend their income. Although others may believe that people with ADHD are unable to realize the long-term effects of their expenses, there is another way to look at the problem: people with ADHD, like people with other disabilities, refuse to recognize the limits of money management. They are less likely to refuse their requests. Of course, it is your responsibility to help your child change his or her behavior.

Nonetheless, when it comes to money, your child will feel helpless. Even if she has her own salary, she obviously relies on you to give her access to money, so you might want to keep an eye on her transactions. You want her to develop financial responsibility and learn to invest on her own, but you still want her to have fun shopping. Finding a comfortable balance isn't always easy.

Without a question, the child's financial activities would have an effect on them. If you waste money irresponsibly, she can imitate your actions. She would never say no to a purchase if she has an infinite supply of cash. She will be unable to invest because money seems to "grow on trees." If you bail her out too much when she doesn't have enough money, she won't learn to save as well. She'll think you'll give her everything in return. And she will be weak and needy if she wishes to be dependent on you.

To foster good financial control, help your child understand that everyone in the household must work under a budget: there is only a limited amount of money available for transactions. And very young children can comprehend this. As soon as your child grasps the concept of "not enough," she will begin to comprehend the concept of inadequate funds.

• Personal Money

Giving personal money to an infant as young as four or five years old has become commonplace. You should keep track of your child's personal money on a sheet of paper so she can see it clearly. It's important to be truthful and give her the money you've set aside without asking. It is beneficial to keep reliable records. It assures her that you are trustworthy, and she begins to learn how to manage a bank account. She'll know how much she will invest and she knows how much money she's saving. Give her the money until you're sure she's ready and understands how to keep it safe and organized.

Offer your child a reward simply for being a member of the family, rather than allowing her to complete a certain task or task (especially if it is not out of the ordinary). The technique eliminates the possibility that if you compensate her, she will refuse to support. It also teaches her how to choose and invest carefully because you'll be asking her to make those transactions with her own capital (e.g. a new doll for her collection). Then you decide what kind of contribution you want her to make from her own money (for example, half the price of the doll).

Emphasize that family members normally support one another without expecting anything in return. If your child's income is unaffected, the family expects she will behave responsibly because it is the "family style." When she isn't acting like that, attempt and figure out why, so don't want to subsidies her if she is acting egotistical and exploiting others.

If you suspect your daughter is scrounging, you might want to reduce her salary. You can openly defend your decisions by saying, "If you don't want to pitch in, we can use your share of the money to hire someone else to help us out." Let her know that the failure to lend a helping hand is the fault of another. Made it clear that you would welcome her participation if she so desired, but it is also necessary to ensure that the household does not function. When a kid continues to steal things from others, loses, or is destructive, it creates a similar dilemma. Make it clear to her that you must keep her accountable in order to protect the interests of others. "We need your funds to help pay for the debt," you might say, and she'll become more conscientious and find less expensive solutions to her irritability. Similarly, if she has a tendency to be reckless in a store, warn her, "Have your bankbook ready for anything that breaks."

• EATING PROBLEMS

You're worried that your child's eating habits will cause her to get embroiled in a scandal she won't want to end. Parents who have children who were born early are constantly in this situation. Their doctors advise them to ensure that their baby loses weight, so they start pushing the baby to feed right away.

Eating will easily turn into a will war. If you want your child to eat well, she must make healthy food decisions. Blocking food entry, using food as a bribe or punishment, attacking her eating habits, using food to distract her, or pressuring her to consume those foods may seem to fix the issue on the surface. Overeating, sneaking food, refusing to eat, and competing for power can all increase as a result of such parenting habits. You might end up leading to atypical eating habits rather than reducing them.

• Solutions

Make it a family tradition to eat at a table together and deem your child's presence at mealtime a pleasure. You don't want to make food an unpleasant experience for yourself. But don't make her do extra work or ask her to complete anything on her desk. You can cause problems if you act disrespectful or annoyed because she is not interested with the food you cook. So, if she isn't interested in what you've prepared, just pack it up and ask her if she needs to eat it later.

Instead of criticizing the amount she consumes, ask, "What is a good amount for one meal?" This method includes her in decision-making and values her with dignity. When you think she's taking too much and depriving others, ask her to assist you in preparing the meals and dividing the servings.

Help her appreciate the advantages of consuming small servings of certain foods; see how you can determine how many to consume in one sitting. "If you're hungry," you might say, "perhaps we have something better for you to eat." The challenge, as usual, is to devise a strategy that works for all of you, and you can't always control what she puts in her mouth. "You can lead a horse to wine, but you can't make it drink," as the saying goes.

It may also be a means to encourage people to consume well by refusing to bring those ingredients into the kitchen. If it's out of sight, it's out of view. Even when there is bad food to be consumed, you want to make healthier food decisions for your kid. Instead of removing her Halloween treats, which may indicate that she lacks self-control, assist her in finding a rational way to handle the sweets.

"It's better for us to eat these foods first," rather than "You can't eat sugar before you eat the veggies," say when encouraging balanced diet. "Sweets is what we consume if we have a little room left at the top," tell her. "We're all selecting healthy diets first to ensure our bodies get what they need," says one participant.

You will improve her food knowledge by asking for her advice when grocery shopping. She would also be delighted if you prepare food according to her preferences, demonstrating that you are aware of her preferences. Unfortunately, extreme adjustment to picky eating will lead to atypical eating habits that are harmful over time.

• Finicky Eating

Although preparing a special meal for your daughter may be a way to show her how much you care, she may not learn to adjust to what the rest of the family is doing if you are constantly attending to her needs. And that won't support her until she enters the real world. Some individuals, for example, will not be able to "jump through the hoops" for your daughter. It could be uncomfortable for her to eat at a friend's or cousin's place. If you only stick to her small menu of options, you can stop her from trying new foods. It's important to ask these questions.

If you disagree with your child's food choices, one alternative is to let them prepare their own lunch. However, it is important that she cleans up after herself when she takes this course. You might say: "I've already prepared a complete meal for the family. Make yourself a sandwich if you want something special, as long as you clean it up right away." The response makes her question if her complaint was reasonable.

• RISK

When a child is diagnosed with ADHD, he or she is usually very active. However, such elevated levels of operation come with dangers as well as benefits. When "the motor revives," your child can love the thrill, freedom from restrictions, and heightened focus, but the side effect could be harmful. That's what concerns you, particularly when she seems to be suffocating your efforts to shield her. Since there can be serious repercussions if you don't get in her path, it's plain to understand how power dynamics can intensify where children are involved.

You want your daughter to get out of her "bubble" and see the world, but you really don't want her to injure herself. You want her to realize that taking such risks isn't worth it. However, if she thinks you're being overly protective, she might stop listening to you entirely. She can become territorial and dig in her heels if she thinks you're threatening her because you don't believe she will win. As a result, walk quietly.

Despite the fact that your daughter has difficulty comprehending the full meaning of her behavior, she understands that you're saying no. So, what's stopping her from talking to you? If you want to keep her safe, you'll have to be incredibly careful before you can fix the dilemma. Sure, you can attempt to ban her and physically restrain her, but it might not always be possible.

• Curbing Risk

No one wants their parents to avoid being involved, so make it clear that you care for her as you encourage caution. Keep in mind that the safety issues often stem from the world's lack of predictability, not from their level of competence. Before you learn more about a situation, tell her you enjoy "keeping it safe." Please inform her "Are you going to assist me in carefully figuring out how to do this?"

• Resolving Resistance

Even with your best intentions, breaking down resistance to

protection demands can be challenging, particularly if siblings or peers have different boundaries. Your daughter, for example, may not choose to wear a cycling helmet if she sees her friends not wearing one. She may be worried about being bullied. This could deter her from protecting herself, as well as her willingness to follow your sound advice. "What do you think of teasing?" ask her if anything happens. If others begin to mock her, attempt to assist her in coming up with a response. The aim is to make your child happier while also emphasizing the advantages of the recommended safety measure. Her follow-up will be suspect until something is done. You might ask her, in order to raise "buy-in," "Why do you think people [use a hat, wear protective glasses, etc.] while they do this activity?" She may be more likely to take the initiative if she understands the benefits for herself.

CONCLUSION

People who are parents or would be parents have thoughts and doubts about how to raise their children. They'll probably want to learn more about what can and shouldn't be done when constructing structures for children of all ages. Raising children is a safe investment for someone who wishes to learn more about being a mother or father, and it can provide you with many benefits.

Many child-raising recommendations are based on child guidelines. Proper development is emphasized because it determines how the children can learn and how well their cognitive and interpersonal abilities will improve. Many science research and parenting books, for example, claim that children learn better and are more likely to be intelligent if they are introduced to music and art at an early age, even while still in their mother's womb. The childcare book will go into how to teach boys and girls about art and music, as well as what kinds of music will aid in growth and learning and other factors that will benefit children's development.

Another main topic in parenting books is nutrition, which has an effect on children's physical and mental growth. Your children would need sufficient nutrition to sustain their bodies and to aid in their development into healthy individuals that are more resistant to viruses and diseases. Since the right kind of food contributes to brain functioning, proper diet has an impact on psychological growth. The childcare guide includes a list of mom and dad's dietary foods that are appropriate for children of all ages and contain additional minerals and vitamins. Furthermore, childcare books will include the kinds of foods that can be avoided or prohibited.

This approach will help parents help their children become more competitive in school, learn more, and be more cooperative at home whether their child has ADHD or is unable to work on it. Note to teachers: some of these techniques will fit in the classroom as well. You will definitely recommend them to parents. Remind him that while he is busy, he must remain in the workplace. This implies that it would concentrate on the following activities: dreaming, reading, writing, and chatting.

Medication for attention deficit hyperactivity disorder. If all methods fail and your child struggles to remain concentrated, your doctor will suggest therapy. The rise can be significant with the right option and dose. However, make sure you talk to a doctor who is experienced with ADHD stimulant medications. The majority of pediatricians do not get much neuropsychopharmacology instruction. Request a referral to a pediatric psychiatrist. You want to ensure that your child receives the proper treatment and the correct dosage.

Diet for ADHD. Food may have unanticipated consequences for infants. Consult the doctor if you believe your diet is causing you problems. Ascertain that your child consumes nutritious foods. Many foods contain sugar and refined protein and are insufficient to cause your child to behave in the manner you suspect he has ADHD. You must consume a nutritious meal.

Select one of these methods at this time. Allow your child to choose the one they like best, as parents are good at introducing children to new things. In phases, add other activities to the list. You'll quickly figure out what works and what doesn't. Teacher, you can select one of two school-based interventions to assist children with ADHD in your class.

Children will, in most situations, ask their own questions and do so for the last time. Stubbornness is a fine indicator of unfavorable activity in every age group's normal context. Guidelines for childcare will teach you how to use verification methods to combat insults and reduce certain habits.

However, there are a number of troubling characteristics and patterns that must be discussed as quickly as possible, and fathers and mothers must use age-appropriate approaches for their infants. Independence, bullying, assaults, and insults are not recommended; child coaching recommendations can explain how to prevent unsafe scenarios like these, as well as how to deal with them if they occur.

Child coaching books, of course, look at exceptional behavior and how to learn to know your girls and boys as they follow your rules and do what they are supposed to do. Responsibility is a type of constructive behavior that both children and mothers of their children want and demonstrate. Suggestion: Child development guides typically do what fathers and mothers need to learn how to be responsible, particularly while their children are present. And as adults, their sons and daughters will be able to understand and express themselves as a result of this. As deeds that will advance accountability, make sure boys and girls build themselves up, do homework from time to time, clean their rooms, and care for dogs.

All has self-esteem, and children must learn to grow it at a young age. When they enter school and make friends with other girls and boys, they will have more confidence and a sense of themselves. Furthermore, both boys and girls were found to be healthier, on social, and more successful in daily life.

Simply put, the parenting guide is intended to assist you in learning more about parenting, how to plan for it, and what to expect from the most difficult work you would ever have.

Parenting an ADHD kid can improve with experience and patience. Don't get frustrated that your child's conduct isn't a sign of your parenting abilities. Adjust your parenting approach to help your child cope with his impulsivity, inattentiveness, and defiance with this in mind.

Be kind to your child, but also to yourselves. Good luck!

Thank you for reading This book.

If you enjoyed it please visit the site where you purchased it and write a brief review. Your feedback is important to me and will help other readers decide whether to read the book too.

Thank you!

Laurel Nash

Want more?

Here is a **free version** of

"The Teenage Mind: A Complete Guide for Parents to Raise Teens With Anxiety, Teaching Them How to Control Anger and Manage Emotions"

Scan the QR-Code!

THE TEENAGE MIND

A Complete Guide for Parents

to Raise Teens With Anxiety, Teaching Them How to Control Anger and Manage Emotions

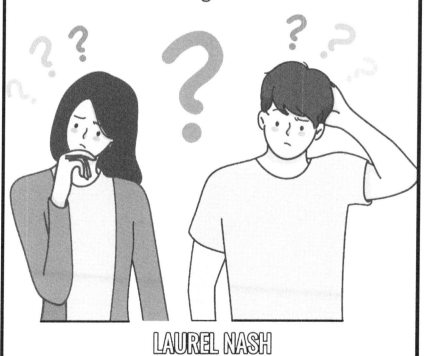

LAUREL NASH

Made in the USA
Coppell, TX
10 October 2021